Questions for Freud

Questions
for
Freud

The Secret History of Psychoanalysis

Nicholas Rand & Maria Torok

Harvard University Press
Cambridge, Massachusetts
London, England
1997

Library of Congress Cataloging-in-Publication Data

Rand, Nicholas T. (Nicholas Thomas)
[Questions à Freud. English]
Questions for Freud : the secret history of psychoanalysis / Nicholas Rand and
Maria Torok.
p. cm.
Includes bibliographical references and index.
ISBN 0-674-74325-3 (alk. paper)
1. Psychoanalysis. 2. Psychoanalysis—History.
3. Psychoanalytic interpretation. 4. Freud, Sigmund, 1856–1939.
I. Torok, Maria.
II. Title.
BF175.R2913 1997
150.19'52—dc21   97-15084

To the memory of
Nicolas Abraham
1919–1975

Contents

Contents

IV Gaining Insight into Freud

Preface

Why is it, we ask, that in Freudian psychoanalysis extraordinary vistas of comprehension are at once opened and closed? We have discovered fundamental theoretical, clinical, and institutional paradoxes at the very core of psychoanalysis. The aim of our *Questions for Freud* is to pinpoint the internal contradictions that undermine the potential effectiveness of key aspects of Freudian thought (concerning, for example, dream interpretation, the origins of neurosis, reality, trauma, fantasy, sexual repression, and the psychoanalytic study of literature)—in the hope of finding the source of those contradictions. Showing that Freudian psychoanalysis is inherently paradoxical, we also call for new insight into Freud the man. Using partially unpublished documents and Freud's own dreams, we isolate a major upheaval that shook Freud and his family in 1865. In the final section of the book we address the question of the genesis of psychoanalysis. What role have hidden family traumas played in shaping Freud's psychological investigations, both promoting and impeding them by turns?

We began research on this book (first published in French in 1995) twenty years ago under vastly different political circumstances for psychoanalysis from today's. At that time, the Freudian establishment was still enjoying its heyday of orthodoxy—and we were fighting for the right to criticize, for the freedom to open Freudian psychoanalysis to internal scrutiny. By the time we published the book, the world, at least around Freud, had changed. The pendulum had swung. As in Charles Laughton's film *The Night of the Hunter*, in which one of the characters rouses the townsfolk to lynch the very preacher she has until then adored, some of Freud's staunchest admirers had all but turned on him. Suddenly it appeared as if we had become his defenders—because we were upholding the value of psychoanalysis despite our diagnosis of its fundamental contradictions.

In any case, attackers or defenders, we are bent on transforming the premise of psychoanalytic inquiry because we have come to realize that Freud was just as often working against as for his creation. We have felt for years that psychoanalysis as a theory and as a therapeutic discipline needs to be made aware of its own internal destructive power before it can hope to answer any criticism from without. Today even the ranks of formerly confident psychoanalysts seem to be in disarray. The solution is not to cast about for new ways of presenting the merits or the inevitability of psychoanalysis in our culture and everyday language, but to allow psychoanalysis to engage in a process of maturation. Instead of indulging in self-pity about the ruthless incomprehension of the outside world, all those interested in a future for psychoanalysis need to sift through the recent assaults against it, asking what is valid in them.

If psychoanalysis is ever to have another lease on life, the first point to consider is that Freudianism in its classical form is indeed indefensible. Second, any proposition that psychoanalysis can be a viable field of psychological exploration and therapy must include an explanation (and not merely a justification) of the impostures, the lies and deceits, the dissimulation and secrets, the exclusions and ostracism that have punctuated the rise of Freudianism and the entire history of the psychoanalytic movement. We are certain that if the recently intensified attacks against psychoanalysis have a real foundation, it is not grounded first and foremost on the charges brought thus far: Freud's alleged dishonesty or misconduct with his patients; his self-serving and propagandistic explanations; his willful misrepresentations and doctored evidence; the lack of independent empirical corroboration of his theories; the absence of safeguards in his system against unexamined dogma or arbitrary interpretations; his failure to produce lasting therapeutic results, let alone cures; the tendency to mistake his own obsessions and fantasies for scientific observation and clinical fact. Though serious, none of these charges would be sufficient to annihilate psychoanalysis as some of its opponents may long have wished. Still, psychoanalysis may as well disappear if it is incapable of escaping from oppressive dogma and if, for its survival, it must rely on an organization whose business it is to prevent the revelation of embarrassing clinical, personal, and historical facts or to deny their relevance.

Whether the disappearance of psychoanalysis is a necessary next step is not for us to predict. We argue that Freudian psychoanalysis is at an impasse today not because, deluding itself, it is the means of deluding others, but because its inherent contradictions have effectively prevented it from determining its own aims ever since its inception. Therefore, in our opinion, even the most trenchant attacks on Freudian psychoanalysis have value as the external manifestations of its own internal disharmony. We will let our readers draw their own conclusions. Our aim here is to spark a new debate with and about Freud's texts, to propose an exchange of opposite views from within the body of Freudian psychoanalytic theory and practice.

Acknowledgments

We want to thank Angela von der Lippe for her acquisition of the manuscript for Harvard. Special thanks to the staff of Harvard University Press, in particular William P. Sisler, Elizabeth Knoll, and Camille Smith, whose high standards and warmth have been inspiring. We also wish to acknowledge the valuable professional advice of David Kornacker, formerly head of the French Publishers' Agency in New York.

Many friends and colleagues, among them Eric Adda, Serge Tisseron, Nelly Furman, John Gedo, Elaine Marks, Yvonne Ozzello, and Marian Rothstein, have contributed in various ways to the successful launch of this book in Europe or the United States. We are also grateful to the many reviewers in France, Germany, and Sweden who have honored our work in its French edition.

Parts of the book appeared previously in *Critical Inquiry* 13, no. 2 (1987) and 19, no. 3 (1993).

Last but not least, our thanks go to the University of Wisconsin–Madison for its generous support of Nicholas Rand in the form of an H. I. Romnes Distinguished Research Award, a residential fellowship at the Humanities Research Institute, numerous summer research grants from the Graduate School, and most recently a five-year appointment to the Humanities Research Institute as a Senior Fellow.

Abbreviations

A   Freud, "The Aetiology of Hysteria," SE 3

AT   J. M. Masson, *The Assault on Truth: Freud's Suppression of the Seduction Theory* (New York: Farrar, Straus, and Giroux, 1984)

CF   *The Correspondence of Sigmund Freud and Sándor Ferenczi,* vol. 1: *1908–1914,* ed. Eva Brabant, Ernst Falzeder, and Patrizia Giampieri-Deutsch, trans. Peter Hoffer (Cambridge, Mass.: Harvard University Press, 1993)

CL   *The Complete Letters of Sigmund Freud to Wilhelm Fliess, 1887– 1904,* ed. and trans. J. M. Masson (Cambridge, Mass.: Harvard University Press, 1985)

DDJ   Freud, "Delusions and Dreams in Jensen's 'Gradiva,'" SE 9

FC   Sándor Ferenczi, *Final Contributions to the Problems and Methods of Psychoanalysis,* ed. Michael Balint, trans. Eric Mosbacher (1955; rpt. New York: Brunner Mazel, 1980)

G   Wilhelm Jensen, "Gradiva: A Pompeiian Fancy," in Freud, *Delusion and Dream and Other Essays,* ed. Philip Rieff (Boston: Beacon Press, 1956)

I   *The Interpretation of Dreams,* SE 4

L   *Introductory Lectures on Psycho-Analysis,* SE 16

LW   Ernest Jones, *The Life and Works of Sigmund Freud,* 3 vols. (New York: Basic Books, 1953–1957)

M   Ludwig Marcuse, *Briefe an und von Ludwig Marcuse* [The Correspondence of Ludwig Marcuse] (Zurich: Diogenes, 1975)

MM *Moses and Monotheism,* SE 23

R   "Repression," SE 14

S   Josef Breuer and Sigmund Freud, *Studies on Hysteria,* ed. and trans. James Strachey, SE 2

SE   *The Standard Edition of the Complete Psychological Works of Sigmund Freud,* ed. and trans. James Strachey, 24 vols. (London: Hogarth Press and the Institute of Psycho-Analysis, 1953–1974)

U   "The Unconscious," SE 14

Questions for Freud

Introduction:
Why Question Freud?

In the hope of enhancing the intrinsic potential of psychoanalysis, we are posing a number of questions for Freud. These are not queries by scientists, looking for criteria of verifiability in psychoanalytic theory; neither are they the questions of sociologists or of philosophers who might examine the contribution of Freudianism to an understanding of society or the self. Our questions reflect the interests of the therapist and the committed student of psychoanalysis. This viewpoint cannot allow disciplines other than psychoanalysis to assess its value. However, in the eyes of psychoanalysis itself, Freudian theory appears beset by fundamental contradictions. We shall uncover some of them, not to diminish Freud's achievement but to know and make known its tensions, to suggest the incessant and insidious effects of these tensions in the lives and works of those who psychoanalyze (people, texts, films, and the visual arts) or are themselves being psychoanalyzed.

If the contradictions of Freudian thought are as basic as we claim, how should we react to them? Why not reject Freud's theories out of hand as fundamentally flawed? Should we perhaps try to free ourselves from paradox by starting from the ground up to build a more cohesive system? Can we overlook the discrepancies and continue to envision and practice psychoanalysis in our own personal ways? All of these reactions are quite acceptable, but what we believe matters is not so much the stance—faithfulness or unfaithfulness, complete repudiation, unquestioning adoption or selective use—as our willingness to rethink the very project of psychoanalysis with the full knowledge that Freud's work evolved along self-contradictory lines.

What is the use of exposing rifts in Freud's thought? Does not this type of return to canonical texts merely shut out the post-Freudian development of psychoanalysis and disregard the many non-Freudian approaches to psychotherapy? We wish to study Freudian paradoxes because we find them just as active today as they were a century ago. We also believe that nearly all modern forms of psychotherapy issue from Freud and therefore share at least some of the contradictions of his thought. These contradictions operate with the same force as they did in Freud's own time because of the specific way in which professional psychoanalysis is transmitted. Freudian theory comes down primarily through analysis; the people practicing it are patients first and only later become certified analysts. Let us admit for the sake of argument that undergoing psychoanalysis is the best preparation for understanding other people. However, this kind of teaching runs the risk of perpetuating flaws. And the gravest flaw in this domain is undoubtedly the patient/analyst's difficulty in reflecting freely on the possibility that the premises of Freudian psychoanalysis are contradictory.

We do not want to show that a Freudian idea is erroneous in itself or that another theory, articulated more recently or validated through more broadly based research, would be more correct. If there are flaws, they are not essentially experimental. The contradictions we see arise from the methodological crux of Freudian theory. Many practitioners are still wondering today how important a role the psychoanalysis of real traumas as opposed to fantasies should play in therapy. Freud's vacillation on this fundamental question has affected every aspect of his theory; unknowingly, we still labor under its influence. Our aim is to halt the nearly unconscious transmission of Freudian methodological rifts. These rifts have thrown psychoanalysis into a disarray in which the most far-reaching understanding of the human psyche collides with a singular absence and, yes, even a refusal of understanding.

The paradoxes of psychoanalysis are symptomatic of its founder's psychic life. How did we arrive at this hypothesis, and what conclusions do we draw from it? We are party to the tradition inaugurated by Freud and cannot but adopt an analytic attitude toward him. We therefore raise the question of the deep-seated reasons behind the contrarieties of Freudian thought. We are not content to assert, as others have done, that Freud uses defective logic or that his enterprise is a mere sham, because our psychoanalytic orientation leads us to inquire into the source of meaning, that is, into the often concealed and painful personal sources of meaning, even of paradoxical meaning. We ask: Why did Freud—wittingly or unwittingly—have a high level of tolerance for clinical, theoretical, and institutional contradictions? We propose an answer: Freud constructed his theories of unconscious mental life even while crucial insight into the traumatic aspects of his immediate family's life forever eluded him. If the methodological fissures of psychoanalysis result from Freud's own familial traumas, we no longer have to adopt the contradictions as our own or continue to hand them down dogmatically. We can hope to be free at last from a perplexing psychoanalytic legacy.

It is hard for us to consider the world without Freud. Ideas such as the unconscious, the dream-work, the deep-seated or latent meaning of mental phenomena, the symptomatic symbolization of conflict, among many others, form and leaven our intellectual daily bread. Our emotional and theoretical heritage is unimaginable without Freud's key ideas, such as the importance of the child to an understanding of the adult, the systematic introduction of sexuality into psychic life, civilized morality and its discontents, or the uneasy intersection of sexuality and society. Without all these and other discoveries by Freud, we would be trying to breathe in a vacuum. Yet we have grave reservations about some Freudian theories, such as penis envy in women, the death drive, frustration as a rule of therapy, and the universal Oedipus and castration complexes.

For a long time we have been torn between gratitude to Freud for having ushered us into the mysteries of the psyche and our growing awareness that theoretical as well as clinical difficulties prevent us from giving him our unquestioning loyalty. Among several others, the following questions have emerged: Can we follow Freud even though in 1897 he set out to replace his initial hypothesis of real traumas with a hypothesis of instinctual fantasies? What are we to do when our respect for the idea of psychoanalysis requires our fidelity to Freud's project and yet, at the same time, we are sure that the application of some of his constructs, such as symbolism in dreams or the successive stages of infantile psychosexual development, is ill-advised? For us the solution to this dilemma is to return to Freud's texts in our own personal way and try to grasp why some of his conceptions compel and repel us by turns. In the course of our study, quite to our astonishment, we have found internal rifts throughout Freud's system of thought.

In other words, we have come to view Freudian psychoanalysis as threatened from within because it combines daring, even revolutionary methods of inquiry with a tendency to restrain questions. Freud's greatest discoveries—the importance of the sexual element, the dream-work, the paths of symptom-formation—lead him to clinical and theoretical impasses. An internal demon of sorts is at work here. The most fully productive and most genuinely original of Freud's ideas also seem to ensnare their creator. Ultimately we need to find an answer to the question: Why is it that in Freudian psychoanalysis narrow-minded practices threaten to overwhelm the spirit of openness?

We are returning to classical psychoanalytic themes—the dream, trauma, seduction, reality, fantasy, sexual repression, and psychoanalytic doctrine applied to literature—because the contradictions are not marginal; they involve Freud's most fundamental, most visible, and most frequently studied theories. In examining the paradoxes of basic psychoanalytic ideas, we perceive over and over again that Freudian theory inevitably fractures. The daily work of both analysts and students of psychoanalysis is impaired by this.

Our aim is to measure the individual paradoxes and demonstrate that, taken together, they form a network of mutually exclusive methodological ambivalences within Freud's thought. Our instances of Freudian contradiction all exhibit the same feature: analytic tools affording unique insight are merged with concepts and techniques that block the progress of understanding. We believe that neither the theoreticians nor the practitioners of psychoanalysis have thus far fully grasped the scope and sources of the internal fissures in Freud's edifice. Most analysts have tacitly chosen certain directions of the theory as the legitimate representatives of Freud and Freudianism. We want to restore the situation as it was prior to any such implicit choices, so that we may see the contradictions plainly and discuss them freely, so that they will no longer operate underground, secretly spreading their mystifying effects.

Needless to say, ours is a fundamental critique of Freudian doctrine. We call for a complete renewal of psychoanalysis. We wish to rouse and sustain the efforts of those professionals and scholars who consider it crucial to preserve psychoanalysis but who also realize the necessity of rethinking it from its foundation. However, we differ from critics who gainsay or seek to eliminate Freudianism by turning to nonpsychoanalytic methodologies. Rather than debate the scientific or nonscientific status of psychoanalysis, we propose to apply the standards of internal coherence only, treating Freud's ideas as self-contained entities that stand or fall on the merits of their own consistency. We are convinced that the malaise surrounding Freud's legacy since the early 1950s is not primarily a result of his riding roughshod over scientific standards, but rather a symptom of the deep-seated and pervasive contrarieties of his thought, clinical practices, and institutional organization. Though intensely critical of Freudian doctrine, we remain ardent advocates of the methods of psychoanalysis as a privileged way of understanding human beings and their creations. We maintain that psychoanalysis can contribute fundamental insights, provided that the internal methodological fractures of Freud's thought are recognized so that it becomes clear which facets of Freudian theory (and of its descendants) fully promote—and which endanger—the freedom of psychological inquiry.[1]

I

*Fundamental Contradictions
of Freudian Thought*

Dream Interpretation: Free Association or Universal Symbolism?

We shall quote two series of passages drawn from *The Interpretation of Dreams* and some other works by Freud. These passages indicate a fundamental methodological discrepancy, as Freud seems to be moving in two contrary directions. He attempts to understand dreams based on the dreamer's free associations, and at the same time he provides a catalog of stable and universally applicable meanings or symbolic equations, rendering the dreamer's personal associations superfluous. The Freudian theory of dream interpretation combines an attempt to hear personal meanings with the use of universal symbolism. The search for the unique poetics of individual dreams collides with the restrictions that predetermined interpretations place upon their meaning.

(1A)

The second of the two popular methods . . . might be described as the "decoding" method, since it treats dreams as a kind of cryptography in which each sign can be translated into another sign having a known meaning, in accordance with a fixed key. Suppose, for instance, that I have dreamt of a letter and also of a funeral. If I consult a "dream-book," I find that "letter" must be translated by "trouble" and "funeral" by "betrothal" . . . A thing in a dream means what it recalls to the mind—to the dream-interpreter's mind, it need hardly be said. An insuperable source of arbitrariness and uncertainty arises . . . [Footnote:] The technique which I describe in the pages that follow differs in one essential respect from the ancient method: it imposes the task of interpretation upon the dreamer himself. (I, 97–98)

(1B)

When we have become familiar with the abundant use made of symbolism for representing sexual material in dreams, the question is bound to arise of whether many of these symbols do not occur with a permanently fixed meaning, like the "grammalogues" in shorthand; and we shall feel tempted to draw up a new "dream-book" on the decoding principle. On that point there is this to be said: this symbolism is not peculiar to dreams, but is characteristic of unconscious ideation, in particular among the people, and it is to be found in folklore, and in popular myths, legends, linguistic idioms, proverbial wisdom and current jokes, to a more complete extent than in dreams. (I, 351)

(2A)

In the case of the decoding method everything depends on the trustworthiness of the "key"—the dream book, and of this we have no guarantee. (I, 100)

(2B)

Incidentally, many of the symbols are habitually or almost habitually employed to express the same thing.   (I, 352)

(3A)

My procedure is not so convenient as the popular decoding method which translates any given piece of a dream's content by a fixed key. I, on the contrary, am prepared to find that the same piece of content may conceal a different meaning when it occurs in various people or in various contexts.   (I, 105)

The dream-content, on the other hand, is expressed as it were in a pictographic script, the characters of which have to be transposed individually into the language of the dream-thoughts. If we attempted to read these characters according to their pictorial value . . . we should clearly be led into error. Suppose I have a picture-puzzle, a rebus, in front of me . . . we can only form a proper judgment of the rebus if . . . we try to replace each separate element by a syllable or word that can be represented by that element in some way or other.   (I, 277–278)

Analyses show us . . . a change in the *verbal expression* of the thoughts concerned . . . the outcome of the displacement may in one case be that one element is replaced by another, while the outcome in another case may be that a single element has its *verbal form* replaced by another . . . The advantage, and accordingly the purpose, of such a change jumps to the eyes. A thing that is pictorial is, from the point of view of a dream, a thing that is *capable of being represented:* it can be introduced into a situation . . . A dream-thought is unusable so long as it is expressed in an abstract form; but when once it has been transformed into pictorial language, contrasts and identifications of the kind which the dream-work requires, and which it creates if they are not already present, can be established more easily than before between the new form of expression and the remainder of the mate-rial underlying the dream. . . We may suppose that a good part of the intermediate work done during the formation of a dream, which seeks to reduce the dispersed dream-thoughts to the most succinct and unified expression possi-ble, proceeds along the line of finding appropriate verbal transformations for the individual thoughts. Any one thought, whose form of expression may happen to be fixed for other reasons, will operate in a determinant and selective manner on the possible forms of expression allotted to the other thoughts, and it may do so, perhaps, from the very start—as is the case of writing a poem. . . In a few instances a change of expression of this kind assists dream-condensa-tion even more directly, by finding a form of words which, owing to its ambiguity, is able to give expression to more than one of the dream-thoughts. In this way the whole domain of verbal wit is put at the disposal of the dream-work. There is no need to be astonished at the part played by words in dream-formation. Words, since they are the nodal points of numerous ideas, may be regarded as predes-tined to ambiguity; and the neuroses (e.g. in framing obses-sions and phobias), no less than dreams, make unashamed use of the advantages thus offered by words for purposes of condensation and disguise. (I, 339–341)

(3B)

Steps, ladders or staircases, or, as the case may be, walking up or down them, are representations of the sexual act.

(I, 355)

All elongated objects, such as sticks, tree trunks and umbrellas . . . may stand for the male organ . . . Boxes, cases, chests, cupboards, and ovens represent the uterus, and also hollow objects, ships, and vessels of all kinds. (I, 354)

Children in dreams often stand for genitals; and indeed, both men and women are in the habit of referring to their genitals affectionately as their "little ones." Stekel is right in recognizing a "little brother" as the penis . . . To represent castration symbolically, the dream-work makes use of baldness, hair cutting, falling out of teeth and decapitation. If one of the ordinary symbols for a penis occurs in a dream doubled or multiplied, it is to be regarded as a warding-off of castration. (I, 357)

I shall now append a few examples of the use of these symbols in dreams, with the idea of showing how impossible it becomes to arrive at the interpretation of a dream if one excludes dream-symbolism, and how irresistibly one is driven to accept it in many cases. (I, 359)

Symbolism is perhaps the most remarkable chapter of the theory of dreams. In the first place, since symbols are stable translations, they realize to some extent the ideal of the ancient as well as of the popular interpretation of dreams . . . (L, 151)

Symbols allow us in certain circumstances to interpret a dream without questioning the dreamer, who indeed would in any case have nothing to tell us about the symbol.
(L, 151)

For when, with experience, we have collected enough of these constant renderings, the time comes when we realize that we should in fact have been able to deal with these portions of dream-interpretation from our own knowledge, and that they could really be understood without the dreamer's associations. (L, 150)

(4A)

There is, in the first place, the universality of symbolism in language . . . Moreover, symbolism disregards differences of language; investigation would probably show that it is ubiquitous—the same for all peoples. (MM, 98–99)

(4B)

Indeed, dreams are so closely related to linguistic expression that Ferenczi has truly remarked that every tongue has its own dream-language. It is impossible as a rule to translate a dream into a foreign language . . . (I, 99)

Considered in its broad outlines, the Freudian doctrine of dream interpretation hardly leads one to suspect methodological disparities. Freud postulated that dreams have a meaning that is relevant to the dreamer's psychic life. Dreams are in part incomprehensible to dreamers, hence the need to interpret them, to find their latent meaning and to make this available to dreamers, allowing them access to hitherto unreachable regions of their own psyches, and thereby giving them control over their own house. The form in which the dream appears upon awakening disguises its genuine signification; the dream is a game of hide-and-seek that dreamers play in and with themselves (the wish versus censorship). Dreams provide the "royal road," according to Freud, to uncovering those internal conflicts from which consciousness has backed away (repression).

The originality of Freud's overall understanding of dreams is strengthened by his interpretive premise: dreams are not to be taken at face value. Freud devised specific techniques for reading dreams; the centerpiece of the technique consists in gathering private information (free associations) from dreamers about the manner in which they unwittingly disguise their own deep-seated purpose. Dream interpretation implies then a form of reading that, with the dreamer's help, undoes distortions, expands condensations, puts displacements back in their place, and sets enigmatic visual images into comprehensible words. Freud calls the various processes of deformation the dream-work, collecting under this name the linguistic and formal procedures that initially render the dream's genuine content inaccessible.

The Interpretation of Dreams (1900) underwent continual change. By 1923, when Freud's complete works *(Gesammelte Schriften)* appeared for the first time, he had expanded the original 543 pages of the book by an additional 185 pages. The additions do not constitute revisions, properly speaking, since the text of the first edition is retained in its entirety; rather, there are shifts of emphasis and to some extent complications of the initial theoretical argument. In 1900 Freud considers the essential novelty of his techniques to be the privileged role he gives dreamers in the interpretation of their own dreams. This argument becomes increasingly snarled as Freud introduces, over the period from 1909 to 1914, the idea of universal dream symbolism. Here are two simultaneous and incompatible Freudian positions: dream interpretation requires the dreamer's participation; the interpretation of dreams has no need for the dreamer's contribution.

Rather than being resolved, the contradiction grows more acute over the years with successive editions of *The Interpretation of Dreams* and with Freud's numerous writings elsewhere on the same subject. Thus in the 1914 edition Freud strengthens his initial position, stating that his technique "imposes the task of interpretation upon the dreamer himself" (I, 98) with the result that the dreamer's associations are what allow the dream to acquire its meaning. At the same time, and in sharp disharmony with that point, Freud inserts, also in 1914, a new fifty-page-long section on representation by universal symbolism in dreams. "When we have become familiar with the abundant use made of symbolism for representing sexual material in dreams, the question is bound to arise of whether many of these symbols do not occur with a permanently fixed meaning, like the 'grammalogues' in shorthand; and we shall feel tempted to draw up a new 'dream-book' on the decoding principle" (I, 351). The two diametrically opposed orientations cannot help colliding. On the one hand, Freud wants to connect dreamers with themselves through their personal free association to their dreams; on the other hand, he ushers dreamers into a world of fixed and universal meanings. The juxtaposition of the two methodologies is striking in this passage from *The Introductory Lectures on Psycho-Analysis* (1916): "In this way we obtain constant translations for a number of dream-elements—just as popular 'dream-books' provide them for *everything* that appears in dreams. You will not have forgotten, of course, that when we use our *associative* technique constant replacements of dream-elements never come to light" (L, 150).

Without entering here into the details of the fluctuating proportions of each of these two methodologies in Freud's work between 1900 and 1939, we would like to point out their essential differences. The inquiry into the personal psychic sense of dreams cannot be compatible with reliance on a catalog of invariable and universally valid meanings. The irreducible distinction between the two methods is this: symbolism imposes meanings that (1) are independent of and (2) preexist individual dreamers, and that (3) are not the dreamer's personal creation. The problem reaches well beyond the theoretical contradiction. Once symbolism becomes an option, it can easily influence dreamers and lead them to produce association in support of the expected meaning. A severed tree symbolizes castration, says the interpreter. The dreamer will respond with his implicit approval: Yes, when I was little, a vicious boy attacked me with his jackknife. The analyst will have provoked associations in keeping with his or her use of universal symbolism. Yet castration, the symbolic meaning of a felled tree, may have inhibited the personal association attached to the particular element of the dream. For example, the association may be: our genealogical tree has been impaired, a branch of the family has been shrouded in mystery and gotten lost. Here symbolism may have eclipsed, if not erased, the dreamer's personal context.

We will consider more closely an example of Freud's use of symbolism:

Steps, ladders, staircases, or, as the case may be, walking up or down them are representations of the sexual act . . . A little time ago I heard that a psychologist whose views are somewhat different from ours had remarked to one of us that, when all was said and done, we did undoubtedly exaggerate the hidden sexual significance of dreams: his own commonest dream was of going upstairs, and surely there could not be anything sexual in *that*. We were put on the alert by this objection, and began to turn our attention to the appearance of steps, staircases and ladders in dreams, and were soon in a position to show that staircases (and analogous things) were unquestionably symbols of copulation. It is not hard to discover the basis of the comparison: we come to the top in a series of rhythmical movements and with increasing breathlessness and then, with a few rapid leaps, we can get to the bottom again. Thus the rhythmical pattern of copulation is reproduced in going upstairs. Nor must we omit to bring in the evidence of linguistic usage. It shows us that "mounting" [German "steigen"] is used as a direct equivalent for the sexual act. We speak of a man as a "Steiger" [a mounter] and of "nachsteigen" ["to run after", literally, "to climb after"]. In French the steps on a staircase are called "marches" and "un vieux marcheur" has the same meaning as our "ein alter Steiger" ["an old rake"].

(I, 355)

In this instance, Freud sets up an inventory of dreams with analogous content and goes on to interpret them uniformly with his own key (here a sexual one) without having recourse to the dreamer's spontaneous associations. Freud justifies the fixed and stable meaning of the dream images on two distinct levels. First justification: the rhythm of climbing up and down the stairs resembles coital movements. He obtains the key here by equating two ideas. Second justification: idiomatic expressions in German and French use images of mounting and walking to denote sexual content. Let us take the example of the French idiom *un vieux marcheur* (literally "an old walker"), whose sexual connotation is quite obvious: an old rake or a dirty old man. In the Freudian interpretation, the dream image, a staircase, disguises the expression *un vieux marcheur* in the well-known and conventional sense, hence the dream indirectly refers to sexual intercourse. Very well. There is apparently nothing to object to here. But did Freud not say earlier that popular dream books were useless precisely because "everything depends on the trustworthiness of the 'key'—the dream book, and of this we have no guarantee" (I, 100)?

Despite his categorical rejection, Freud forges his own keys, believing that he is setting them on an unfailingly solid foundation. "The distinction between dream-interpretation of this kind and interpretation by means of symbolism [in popular dream books] can still be drawn quite sharply. In the case of [the popular] symbolic dream-interpretation the key to the symbolization is arbitrarily chosen by the interpreter; whereas in our cases of verbal disguises the keys are generally known and laid down by firmly established linguistic usage" (I, 341). In Freud's eyes, symbolism is justified so long as it relies on meanings established by convention; it seems to follow that accepted meanings are by definition universally valid and applicable to all. But does convention or accepted meaning guarantee the permanent stability of keys? The dream image of going up a steep path, for example, can refer to one's efforts to reach a specific goal or to the toil of life in general. Similarly, a staircase can make us think of delayed reaction (as in the French idiom *avoir l'esprit de l'escalier,* "to be slow with repartee") or, alternatively, of professional incompetence (as in the colloquial French idiom *le coiffeur fait des escaliers dans les cheveux de sa cliente,* literally, "the hairdresser is making staircases in his client's hair"). Freud's technique, reliance on "the evidence of linguistic usage," cannot vouchsafe a dream's permanent symbolic meaning.

If psychoanalysis has any authority at all, in our opinion, it is the willingness to welcome people into their own personal creations. And quite often Freud did not think otherwise. But just as often he sought to found the authority of psychoanalysis on universally accepted forms of expression. "Symbolism is not peculiar to dreams, but is characteristic of unconscious ideation . . . and it is to be found in folklore, and in popular myths, legends, linguistic idioms, proverbial wisdom and current jokes, to a more complete extent than in dreams" (I, 351). So the dream image showing a man climbing the stairs is said to be reliably translated every time, with the help of the common French idiom *un vieux marcheur,* as a dream of coitus. In sum, Freud hoped to draw up a universally trustworthy glossary of conventional meanings or symbols. Here we must raise the fundamental question: Is Freud attempting to reveal by dream analysis the dreamer's inalienable and personal psychic patrimony, or to recover a historical, cultural, and linguistic heritage that is allegedly known and commonly used by all? Is it possible to maintain that personal meanings coincide with universal ones?

Consider the dream image of a man walking along a path and

the attendant free association that focuses on the French expression *un vieux marcheur.* The psychoanalytic procedure need not seize upon the conventional use of this expression as the center of the entire explanation of the dream. This would be tantamount to declaring the idiom a ready-made sexual key, a procedure that might compromise our understanding of the dreamer's personal situation—perhaps, in this case, entirely devoid of sexual overtones. Listening to more of the associations, the analyst may begin to wonder: Who is being called a *vieux marcheur?* Under what circumstances? Why is the dreamer using precisely this characterization when speaking of his dream? Despite its obvious conventional meaning, does the idiom have to be broken down into its constituent parts? What does it mean for the dreamer to walk or not to walk?

The situation emerges little by little. For a long time, the patient has participated in an arrangement *(un vieux marcheur)* he now wants to back out of. Years ago, he let himself be included in a secret agreement he no longer wishes to honor. The dream marks a turning point; the dreamer reviews his entire life on this occasion. The expression *un vieux marcheur* signals an internal and nearly conscious exclamation, I will no longer go along with this kind of arrangement! The pejorative irony of the term *un vieux marcheur* underscores the patient's self-criticism as regards his own past. The complete individual meaning of the dream image showing a man walking along a path and of the free association to *un vieux marcheur* can be rendered as follows: I sense that I am no longer going to follow that path; I renege on this shady old agreement; I am going to set out on a new path.

Though seemingly firm in his embrace of symbolism, Freud is not undisturbed by questions. Discussing the issue of verbal ambiguity as used in dreams (see quotation 3A above), Freud wonders, without providing an answer, whether a dream element "is to be interpreted symbolically" or whether "its interpretation is to depend on its wording" (I, 341). Freud vacillates between

20

the two interpretive viewpoints, but his hesitation seems to us unjustified on the theoretical level. The method that relies on permanent symbolic keys is inadequate to decipher the verbal and affective distortions of a dream's unique, individual meaning. What matters in psychoanalysis is not the evidence of language or of cultural traditions and their customary forms of expression but each person's distinctive signification. The analyst may not subordinate the patient to the accepted, conventional meaning of a set idiom; rather, idioms need to be adapted to what patients are trying to express through them. The analyst's task is to listen to patients, not to situate them in the preconceived field of universal symbolism.

Throughout his long career, Freud rejected, accepted, and nuanced by turns the use of symbolism in dream interpretation. He eschewed its arbitrariness, and yet he would have liked to translate dreams into a stable, authentic, and indisputably universal code. In the successive editions of *The Interpretation of Dreams,* Freud tended to reinforce the authority of symbolism, and yet—here is the crux of the discrepancy—he did not diminish the significance of his discoveries concerning the unique expressive procedures to be found in individual dreams. From 1909 on he laid ever more emphasis on the links between dreams and what he called primeval modes of expression, prevalent in archaic societies. Symbolism seemed to Freud to be the relic of a common archaic heritage—this is why he thought he could certify the universal validity of dream symbolism. "We may expect that the analysis of dreams will lead us to a knowledge of man's archaic heritage, of what is psychically innate in him. Dreams and neuroses seem to have preserved more mental antiquities than we could have imagined possible; so that psycho-analysis may claim a high place among the sciences which are concerned with the reconstruction of the earliest and most obscure periods of the beginnings of the human race" (I, 549)

Freud assigned two disparate functions to dreams. He attempted to situate them in the continuum of the dreamer's individual mental life, and at the same time he wanted to discover in dreams the remnants of ancient or primitive modes of thinking, a kind of innate mental inheritance. Freud understood his task to be the psychoanalysis of specific human beings through their dreams, but he also wanted to see dreams as the medium through which the remnants of universal mental forms, once characteristic of ancient civilizations, live on every night. Consequently, he tried to join the dreamer's variable personal associations with the generalized and invariable associations provided by symbolism.

In our estimation these two orientations are incompatible. Their combination in *The Interpretation of Dreams* makes it an ambivalent book; Freud's innovations gradually merge with the initially discredited method of interpreting dreams by means of ready-made keys. It is as if in the Freudian doctrine of dream interpretation two contrary principles are made to overlap. With his study of the poetic form of dreams (condensation displacement, representation through composite images, overdetermination, and so on), Freud devised an original method of interpretation on the premise that dreams cannot be taken at face value if they are to yield their latent meanings. Freud was seeking precise analytical tools with which to make sense of apparently senseless or disjointed dreams. This type of inquiry into the dream's modes of expression allows the dreamer unlimited freedom. Yet Freud curtails this freedom. By including symbolism, he establishes fixed characteristics that ultimately restrict the dream's potential field of signification, binding it to a set of predetermined contents.

We have drawn up a partial catalog of Freud's contradictory views on dream interpretation. Some readers will ask whether Freud himself was not aware of the difference between his two methods of analysis, individualized interpretation with the aid of free association and fixed translations through universal symbols. We respond that Freud was undoubtedly aware of the diversity of approaches; several passages in *The Interpretation of Dreams* and the *Introductory Lectures on Psycho-Analysis* make this quite plain. However, Freud did not draw the necessary logical conclusion, namely that the two modes of interpretation are mutually exclusive. His desire to combine them seems inexplicable to us, since it leads to a fundamental incompatibility that debilitates all of psychoanalytic theory and practice. Those who may think that other works by Freud resolve the methodological paradoxes of dream interpretation will only find more paradoxes—and no way out. It is up to Freud's followers to resolve his contradictions, after first recognizing them as such.[1]

The Concept of Psychical Reality
and Its Traps

We are studying internal rifts in Freudian psychoanalysis. The methodological paradox of dream interpretation seems to us typical, although others will undoubtedly see it as an exception. However, as we uncover yet another area of Freud's vacillation, this time between the lived reality of sexual traumas and the instinctual fantasies, it will become clear that equally basic contradictions inhere in Freud's inquiries into the laws of psychopathology.

Freud defined the concept of psychical reality in 1916 in the twenty-third of his *Introductory Lectures on Psycho-Analysis*. The idea of a category of reality—in this instance, fantasy—obtaining only in the psychological realm would appear to signal a major step forward in Freud's attempts to delimit the mechanisms of mental life. But this is not entirely the case. The idea of psychical reality overlaps with and serves to mask the inherent contradiction of a question that was to trouble Freud throughout his career: Is what patients say about their childhood experiences true or false? Freud's dilemma, as we see it, consisted in his being unwilling and perhaps unable to determine the real or fantasized status of his patients' accounts. The result is an odd dilemma: Freud does not seem to know with certainty what he is working on as an analyst—truth or lies, traumas or fantasies? That question is raised, whether directly or indirectly, with persistence between 1896 and 1932, and Freud's answer is less than satisfying: he responds with a *non liquet:* there is doubt, it is never quite clear or certain.[2]

With the concept of psychical reality Freud appears to be asserting the independence or, even more forcefully, the autonomy of mental phenomena as regards external and objective reality. The psychic realm has its own laws, wholly unknown to other domains. Mental productions, foremost among them fantasy, belong to a realm in which reality and imagination, truth and lie intermingle, are interchangeable, because the features of this mental universe differ fundamentally from those of the objective world. Fantasy and reality may coexist, can even replace each other—this is, in 1916, Freud's view of the specificity of mental life as manifested in the neuroses. Freud isolates three kinds of typical occurrences in childhood—observation of parental intercourse, seduction by an adult, and the threat of being castrated—noting that in these cases it would be pointless to try to ascertain veracity or falsehood. Whether these "essential elements of a neurosis" (Freud) derive from real events or from fantasy is irrelevant. The outcome will be the same in both cases, since lived reality of external events and imaginary fantasies lead to identical neurotic effects. A theory of the psyche according to which only effects, and not their real or imagined sources, are judged to be of consequence seems so coherent and rigorous that we tend to overlook its paradoxical antecedents in Freud's thought.

Freud raised the question of truth and fiction, that is, of infantile sexual traumas versus fantasies of seduction, in the most acute of terms on 21 September 1897 when, in a letter to his friend Wilhelm Fliess, he announced his abandonment of the hypothesis of infantile seduction as the cause of adult hysteria. In the letter Freud asserts that it is impossible to distinguish between truth and fiction in the unconscious and wonders whether the scenes of seduction, reconstructed up to that point in psycho-analysis and assumed to be genuine, were not instead mere sexual fantasies. This crisis—apparently resolved in the same month, September 1897, with Freud's reversal of his own theory of the reality of early traumas, but in fact never fully resolved—delineates one of the most fundamental contradictions in Freudian theory. It is crucial to understand the full extent of this contradiction between truth and falsehood because it has subtly made its way into Freud's contemporary legacy, threatening even now to disrupt the progress of psychoanalytic listening and understanding. Bringing to light Freud's long-term vacillation is all the more pressing as most interested readers and even Freud specialists have endorsed the idea of his swift and definitive repudiation of the seduction theory. After showing the scope of Freud's etiological vacillation, we will need to ask why Freud could not break from the choice between reality and fantasy, truth versus fiction and lies. Why did he wonder so strenuously whether what his patients told him was true or false?

Much ink has already been spilled over Freud's disavowal of the seduction theory. Is it really necessary to treat the subject yet again? Definitely yes. No matter how far we advance the date of Freud's retraction of the seduction theory beyond the commonly accepted year of 1897, we keep finding clues that undermine the firmness of his initial renunciation. Evidence suggests that Freud did not simply face a choice—seduction or fantasy—but that he was permanently of two minds.

Events of this sort strengthen our impression that the patients must really have experienced what they reproduce under the compulsion of analysis as scenes from their child-hood. But another and stronger proof of this is furnished by the relationship of the infantile scenes to the content of the whole of the rest of the case history. It is exactly like putting together a child's picture-puzzle: after many at-tempts, we become absolutely certain in the end which piece belongs in the empty gap; for only that one piece fills out the picture and at the same time allows its irregular edges to be fitted into the edges of the other pieces in such a manner as to leave no free space and to entail no overlap-ping. In the same way, the contents of the infantile scenes turn out to be indispensable supplements to the associative and logical framework of the neurosis, whose insertion makes its course of development for the first time evident, or even, as we might often say, self-evident.   (A, 205)

Prior to the crisis of 1897 Freud exerted as much persuasive energy to demonstrate the authenticity of infantile scenes of se-duction as he was to use later to show the opposite. Thus he wrote in 1924:

Before going further into the question of infantile sexuality I must mention an error into which I fell for a while and which might well have had fatal consequences for the whole of my work. Under the influence of the technical procedure which I used at that time, the majority of my patients reproduced from their childhood scenes in which they were sexually seduced by some grown-up person . . . I believed these stories, and consequently supposed that I had discov-ered the roots of the subsequent neurosis in these experi-ences of sexual seduction in childhood. . . When, however, I was at last obliged to recognize that these scenes of seduc-tion had never taken place, and that they were only fantasies which my patients had made up or which I myself had

perhaps forced on them, I was for some time completely at
a loss . . . When I had pulled myself together, I was able to
draw the right conclusions from my discovery: namely, that
the neurotic symptoms were not related directly to actual
events but to wishful phantasies, and that as far as the
neurosis was concerned psychical reality was of more importance than material reality.

(*An Autobiographical Study*, SE 20:33–34)

And in 1914 he wrote:

Analysis had led back to these infantile sexual traumas by
the right path, and yet they were not true. The firm ground
of reality was gone. . . If hysterical subjects trace back their
symptoms to traumas that are fictitious, then the new fact
which emerges is precisely that they create such scenes in
phantasy, and this psychical reality requires to be taken into
account alongside practical reality. This reflection was soon
followed by the discovery that these phantasies were intended to cover up the autoerotic activity of the first years
of childhood, to embellish it and raise it to a higher plane.
And now, from behind the phantasies, the whole range of a
child's sexual life came to light.

(*On the History of the Psycho-Analytic Movement*, SE 14: 17–18)

The strength of Freud's conviction of the fictitious nature of
infantile seduction scenes is matched only by the intensity of his
earlier belief in their reality. In 1896, in the synthetic article
entitled "The Aetiology of Hysteria," Freud lists no fewer than
nine proofs in support of the genuineness of these scenes. One
of them seems to him "to provide conclusive proof" (A, 204)
since, despite the most convincing reproduction of their experiences, it is the patients themselves who "still attempt to withhold
belief" (A, 204). "This latter piece of behaviour seems to provide

conclusive proof. Why should patients assure me so emphatically of their unbelief, if what they want to discredit is something which—from whatever motive—they themselves have invented?" (A, 204).

Freud later thought he had found the motive—instinctually determined fantasies—and could confirm its validity beyond doubt. However, as he was preparing to reprint his early essay of 1896 in 1924, he added a highly ambiguous footnote at the conclusion of the series of proofs he had marshaled in favor of the reality of seduction scenes. "All this is true; but it must be remembered that at the time I wrote it I had not yet freed myself from my *overvaluation* of reality and my *low valuation* of phantasy" (A, 204). Given its relatively late date, this footnote is perplexing. What is true, the genuineness of seduction scenes or their fictitious nature? Or perhaps both are true, side by side, with the full weight of the contradiction this juxtaposition implies. At first glance there is no inconsistency. After all, researchers have the right to reverse themselves if their results so require. The whole problem would have ceased to exist were it not for the fact that Freud never definitively relinquished his seduction theory despite his forceful repudiation of it. If the date of the footnote in question were not 1924, a period in which Freud was producing the masterly works of his maturity and a time when the old seduction theory seemed to have been long superseded, there would be no cause for surprise. Yet this kind of surprise—a hesitancy concerning the real or imagined ground of neurotic symptoms—awaits Freud's readers at unforeseeable intervals from 1897 on until 1924, if not well beyond.

Freud's initial turmoil, following the retraction of a clinical discovery he no doubt cherished, is quite evident in his letters to Fliess but has been obscured by commentators. Ever since the publication in 1985 of *The Complete Letters of Sigmund Freud to Wilhelm Fliess*, there can be no doubt that Freud zigzagged, sometimes to the point of bewilderment (in his own words), between the old and the new theory. In order to appreciate the painful intensity of Freud's vacillation, it is necessary to review his letters from the relevant period (1897–1900) in detail.

Freud's oscillations recurred in cycles throughout the entire period of his conceptual gestation (1897–1900), seeming to restore the primacy of "seduction" just as "fantasy" was gaining the upper hand. However, these are not lasting reversions to the former theory; no sooner does "seduction" reappear—as if it had never left the clinical scene—than it is once more thrust aside in favor of "fantasy." Freud's vacillation can be followed systematically in his private correspondence with Fliess as well as in "Screen Memories," an essay he published in 1899. In our discussion we will privilege quotations pertaining to the recurrences of the seduction theory, because these passages are virtually unknown, whereas the development of the theory of instinctual fantasies is widely disseminated, its outlines in the Freud-Fliess letters having enjoyed a prominent place for nearly half a century in both the scholarly and the popular accounts of Freudian doctrine.[3]

A few months after his retraction of the seduction theory (seduction by the father, among other adults), Freud wrote to Fliess on 12 December 1897: "My confidence in paternal etiology has risen greatly. Eckstein deliberately treated her patient in such a manner as not to give her the slightest hint of what would emerge from the unconscious and in the process obtained from her, among other things, the identical scenes with the father" (CL, 286). Soon thereafter, on 22 December, the abandoned theory resurfaced once more; seduction reappears in the long description (printed in full in Chapter 6) of a case of paternal child abuse: "The intrinsic authenticity of infantile trauma is borne out by the following little incident . . ." (CL, 288). This same letter includes a new motto Freud was planning for his study of hysteria: "What have they done to you, poor child?" The motto was to have confirmed Freud's renewed confidence in his previously rejected theory.

A year after the disavowal, a year dominated by the hypothesis of sexual fantasy, Freud speaks, on 31 August 1898, of his etiological bewilderment, quoting an adage to describe his contradictory state: "The way to gain riches, according to an apparently eccentric but wise saying, is to sell your last shirt. The secret of this restlessness is hysteria. In the inactivity here and in the absence of any fascinating novelty, the whole business has come to weigh heavily on my soul. My work now appears to me to have far less value, and my disorientation to be complete . . ." (CL, 325). A month later, on 27 September, we see the dilemma turning into rumination: "Now, a child who regularly wets his bed until his seventh year (without being epileptic or the like) must have experienced sexual excitation in his earlier childhood. Spontaneous[ly] or by seduction? There it is . . . You see, if need be, I could say to myself, 'It is true I am cleverer than all the coxcombs. . .,' but the sad sentence that follows does not fail to apply to me either: 'I lead my people around by the nose and see that we can know nothing'" (CL, 329).

With the new year the question seems temporarily resolved. On 3 January 1899 every hesitation is, for a brief interval at least, "definitively" put to rest: "In the first place, a small bit of my self-analysis has forced its way through and confirmed that fantasies are products of later periods and are projected back from what was then the present into earliest childhood . . . To the question 'What happened in earliest childhood?' the answer is 'Nothing, but the germ of a sexual impulse existed'" (CL, 338). Later that same month, 30 January 1899, Freud goes so far as to speak confidently of "fantasy as the key": "Puberty is becoming ever more central; fantasy as the key holds fast" (CL, 342).

Paradoxe oblige, but we half expected it: the security afforded by the etiological certainty of fantasy will be short-lived. After nine months of relative calm, the abandoned seduction theory makes yet another forceful comeback. In the letter dated 21 December 1899 we read:

> I am not without one happy prospect. You are familiar with my dream which obstinately promises the end of E's treatment (among the absurd dreams), and you can well imagine how important this one persistent patient has become to me. It now appears that the dream will be fulfilled. I cautiously say "appears," but I am really quite certain. Buried deep beneath all his fantasies, we found a scene from his primal period (before twenty-two months) which meets all the requirements and in which all the remaining puzzles converge. It is everything at the same time—sexual, innocent, natural, and the rest. I scarcely dare believe it yet. It is as if Schliemann had once more excavated Troy, which had hitherto been deemed a fable. At the same time the fellow is doing outrageously well. He demonstrated the reality of my theory in my own case, providing me in a surprising reversal with the solution, which I had overlooked, to my former railroad phobia. For this piece of work I even made him the present of a picture of Oedipus and the Sphinx.
>
> (CL, 391–392)

With this letter of 21 December 1899 Freud excavates the infantile seduction scenes that since 1897 he has wanted to consider as mere fables, and, like a second Schliemann, he once again pronounces them truthful. Freud's reversion to the reality of infantile scenes—for which the letter of 21 December 1899 provides an all but triumphant witness—is temporary; it is quickly overshadowed by depression and a sense of helplessness. On 11 March 1900 Freud speaks again in the following terms:

> For my second iron in the fire is after all my work—the prospect of reaching an end somewhere, resolving many

doubts, and then knowing what to think of the chances of my therapy. Prospects seemed most favorable in E.'s case—and that is where I was dealt the heaviest blow. Just when I believed I had the solution in my grasp, it eluded me and I found myself forced to turn everything around and put it together anew, in the process of which I lost everything that until then had appeared plausible. I could not stand the depression that followed. Moreover, I soon found that it was impossible to continue the really difficult work in a state of mild depression and lurking doubts. When I am not cheerful and collected, every single one of my patients is my tormentor. I really believed I would have to give up on the spot. I found a way out by renouncing all conscious mental activity so as to grope blindly among my riddles. Since then I am working perhaps more skillfully than ever before, but I do not really know what I am doing. I could not give an account of how matters stand. (CL, 403–404)

The new century opens with a veritable crisis for Freud. His constant shifts of direction, his erratic changes of heart—first abandoning the seduction theory, then putting it back into service, only to reject it once again—all of this leaves Freud disconcerted. No matter how hard he tries, he can neither fully embrace nor definitively renounce his first theory of neurosis, real sexual seduction in childhood. As a result, his new hypothesis, seduction as fantasy, is not stable by 1900, much less consolidated. The pithiest and most striking manifestation of Freud's theoretical vacillation takes place in his essay "Screen Memories" (1899). The same controversy as in the private correspondence rages between the authenticity of infantile recollections and the role of sexual fantasies. The essay is a dramatization of the internal debate; as in a play, two interlocutors represent opposite points of view. It is Freud's own internal debate concerning the authenticity of infantile scenes, a debate he carries out in public. The essay ends on a note of characteristic indecision—"with no concern for historical accuracy" (SE 3: 322)—after providing the reader with conceptual proof both for and against the idea that instinctual fantasies lurk behind real or imaginary if not outright false recollections. By its dual nature, the concept of screen memory aptly designates the persistence of two opposite views in Freud's thinking at the turn of the century, a period when, if we believe the historians and commentators of psychoanalysis, one of the two conceptions had long prevailed and now held exclusive sway over Freud's thought.

For his definition of screen memory, a term he invented, Freud relied on the work of two French psychologists, V. and C. Henri, concerning the vicissitudes of memory as regards the events of childhood. Freud linked the Henri brothers' findings with his own investigations, dating back to the period of his collaboration with Josef Breuer, on the pathological amnesia of hysterics who have no access to their memory of traumatic events (that is, the lost memory of lived experiences whose recollection would help to alleviate their suffering). Freud used and refined the Henris' observations that insignificant recollections from childhood cover up and sometimes distort the authentic memory of "serious and tragic events" (ibid., 305). Erasing the effects of distortion, displacement, and omission—in a word, doing away with the screen memory in order to recover the repressed recollection of traumatic events—defines the aim of psychoanalytic therapy as Freud advocated it in 1899.

Yet, at the same time, and running counter to that idea, Freud discusses another category of screen memories, the category of falsified recollection, screening out not an authentic memory but an underlying unconscious fantasy. Two lines of thought intersect in the essay: (1) a trivial memory displaces the repressed recollection of a truly important and often traumatic event; (2) the recollection is false as such and stands in the way of a forgotten or unacknowledged fantasy. These two conceptions are antagonistic if we credit Freud's subsequent account of his theoretical development (see the passages quoted above from 1914 and 1924). However, in analyzing his own screen memory, Freud stages a fictitious dialogue between opponents who both represent him. Over his partner's vehement objections, Freud pleads for the indisputable genuineness of memories from childhood, even as he also sees in these recollections of real events a false screen for sexual fantasies. Freud ends the century vacillating; he continues to tussle between truth and falsehood, between the genuine recollection and the fantasy of childhood scenes.

In spite of what he had hoped and what he subsequently said, Freud was not at peace with this problem during the new century. The nagging qualms about truth and falsehood, fantasy and seduction do not stop resounding in his works. Perhaps for want of a friend in whom to confide his clinical and theoretical second thoughts, Freud no longer treats his doubt with the pathos we see in his letters to Fliess. In fact, Freud does not even recognize his doubts as a problem. Yet neither the pathos nor his doubts have disappeared, though the vacillations take on a much less direct form, haunting, as it were, his writings and theoretical elaborations.

What astonishes us most is that the considerable theoretical advances of Freudian thought at the start of the twentieth century should not have succeeded in neutralizing the question of truth and falsehood in Freud's mind. The light he shed on infantile sexuality, the role of the stages of instinctual and libidinal development in the neuroses, the pathogenic importance of repressed unconscious fantasies, as related in particular to the Oedipus complex—all the new theories, which in the eyes of nearly everyone defined the quintessence of psychoanalysis, failed to satisfy Freud. These elaborations failed to quiet in him the turmoil of the choice between truth and falsehood.

And yet, whether we adhere to them or not, Freud's mature

theories clearly lay claim to a level of cohesiveness and universal validity that no longer requires a return to the question of truth versus falsehood. Nobody but Freud requires it. Most of his disciples will have had little trouble in embracing the views that flourished after the *Three Essays on the Theory of Sexuality* (1905). Moreover, classical Freudian psychoanalysis continues to this day to center on ideas concerning the vicissitudes of psychosexuality. As Freud continually perfected his conceptions, adding new ones such as narcissism, the second theory of the instincts (life and death instincts), the superego, the basis remained unchanged for his disciples. The theory of the instincts cemented the whole edifice. But the cement that, in the eyes of others, joins Freud's doctrines, proved insufficiently solid in his own eyes. The question of the reality of the sexual events of childhood, no doubt long laid to rest for others, was not closed for Freud.

In 1908, as new and nearly definitive form was being given to hysteria in the essay "Hysterical Phantasies and Their Relation to Bisexuality," Freud's vacillation persisted. Defining hysteria as being due to the conversion of unconscious sexual fantasies into symptoms, Freud interrupts his discussion to add definitions of hysteria that throw him back to some fifteen years earlier: "Hysterical symptoms are mnemic symbols of certain operative (traumatic) impressions and experiences. Hysterical symptoms are substitutes, produced by conversion, for the associative return of these traumatic experiences" (SE 9: 163). In a startling statement, Freud says that these differing points of view "do not contradict each other" (ibid.). This is the more misleading as we know how hard he worked to demonstrate the opposition of these very viewpoints. The passages from 1914 and 1924 (quoted in full earlier) bear witness: "Analysis had led back to these infantile sexual traumas by the right path, and yet they were not true. The firm ground of reality was gone" (1914). "I was at last obliged to recognize that these scenes of seduction had never taken place, and that they were only phantasies which my patients had made up" (1924). The paradoxical amalgamation of the two contraries passes almost unnoticed in a text from 1913, "The Claims of Psycho-Analysis to Scientific Interest": "psycho-analysis has shown that they [symptoms] are mimetic representations of scenes (whether actually experienced or only invented) *[von er-lebten und gedichteten Szenen]* with which the patient's imagination is occupied without his becoming conscious of them" (SE 13: 172–173).

From 1897 on Freud shackled himself with the question of truth versus falsehood without ever examining its ultimate meaning or his own reasons for the interrogation. The question survives with the old intensity well into 1916–1917, in the most systematic and the most influential of Freud's general accounts of his discoveries, for example in the *Introductory Lectures on Psycho-Analysis* and *From the History of an Infantile Neurosis* (the case of the Wolf Man). We see in this continuing tenacity of the question of truth versus falsehood (especially during this period of the magisterial consolidation of psychoanalytic theory) a reflection of Freud's own intimate personality. Keeping this question alive—even though it had long been superseded in actual fact and rendered obsolete by the psychoanalytic inquiries of the day—signals to us an inner suffering on Freud's part. We will later ask why Freud came to doubt the veracity of the traumatic events related by his patients and why he thought he could identify lies in their accounts. For the moment we will consider briefly the last major instance of this problem, in order to suggest the type of clinical and theoretical impasse Freud's vacillation concerning reality and fantasy implies for the analyst and the student of psychoanalysis.

Because Freud could neither reject nor accept the reality of infantile traumatic sexual events, he emphasized in 1916 the value of a hybrid concept, psychical reality, in which truth and falsehood coincided. It is worth stressing that in Freud's terminology (see the twenty-third of the *Introductory Lectures*) psychical reality does not signify the whole of inner life: "psychical reality" denotes primarily fantasy, that is, the mental productions of infantile realities that later turn out to be false. "It remains a fact that the patient has created these phantasies for himself, and this fact is of scarcely less importance for his neurosis than if he had really experienced what the phantasies contain. The phantasies possess *psychical* as contrasted with *material* reality, and we gradually learn to understand that *in the world of the neuroses it is psychical reality which is the decisive kind*" (L, 368). In short, psychical reality is for Freud the falsification of objective or material reality.

Given this definition, which underscores the absolute opposition between material reality and fantasy, one may wonder what provoked Freud's choice of the term reality (even if psychical) to designate what, in the same lecture, he keeps calling invented stories, fictions, falsehood, and falsified memories. Why does not Freud treat fantasy in the same way as other mental phenomena he had previously studied, dreams, slips of the tongue, affects, symptoms, and the like? Do they not possess an equally autonomous significance and validity within the internal mental world of humans? Is it necessary to set mental phenomena in diametrical contrast to so-called material reality? With the term "psychical reality" Freud asserts one thing and its opposite: "psychical reality" states truth and falsehood at the same time; it amalgamates reality and its falsification.

If after 1913 Freud uses the term "psychical reality" to denote fantasy, it is because he continues to grapple with his own early vacillation between the reality and the falsehood of infantile scenes.

> If the infantile experiences brought to light by analysis were invariably real we should feel that we were standing on firm ground; if they were regularly falsified and revealed as in-

ventions, as phantasies of the patient, we should be obliged to abandon this shaky ground and look for salvation elsewhere. But neither of these things is the case: the position can be shown to be that the childhood experiences constructed or remembered in analysis are sometimes indisputably false and sometimes equally certainly correct, and in most cases compounded of truth and falsehood. Sometimes, then, symptoms represent events which really took place and to which we may attribute an influence on the fixation of the libido, and sometimes they represent phantasies of the patient's which are not, of course, suited to playing an etiological role. It is difficult to find one's way about in this. We can make a first start, perhaps, with a similar discovery— namely, that the isolated childhood memories that people have possessed consciously from time immemorial and before there was any such thing as analysis may equally be falsified or at least may combine truth and falsehood in plenty. In their case there is seldom any difficulty in showing their incorrectness; so we at least have the reassurance of knowing that the responsibility for this unexpected disappointment lies, not with analysis, but in some way with the patients.   (L, 367)

Since Freud cannot decide whether it is a matter of one or the other, reality or fiction, in 1916 he proposes to equate the two, explaining that as far as the patient is concerned it "will be a long time before he can take in our proposal that we should equate phantasy and reality and not bother to begin with whether the childhood experiences under examination are the one or the other. Yet this is clearly the only correct attitude to adopt towards these mental productions" (L, 368).

For a moment it seems as if Freud's new proposition—that material reality and fantasy are indistinguishable in mental life, indeed the distinction between them is useless—will soothe his recurrent vacillation. If it is true, as Freud states, that the "outcome is the same, and up to the present we have not succeeded in pointing to any difference in the consequences, whether phantasy or reality has had the greater share in these events of childhood" (L, 370), then his original question should have lost its relevance. Well, not quite. Freud is visibly unhappy with his definition. No sooner does he establish the absolute primacy of fantasy (psychical reality) than he finds proofs of material reality:

> Among the occurrences which recur again and again in the youthful history of neurotics—which are scarcely ever absent—there are a few of particular importance, which also deserve on that account, I think, to be brought into greater prominence than the rest . . . It would be a mistake to suppose that they are never characterized by material reality; on the contrary, this is often established incontestably through enquiries from older members of the patient's family. (L, 368–369)

It is perhaps with a view to confirming the hypothesis of some ultimate reality that Freud finally conjectures a new category of fantasy—primal fantasies—the contemporary descendants of a long-gone material reality: "In them the individual reaches beyond his own experience into primaeval experience . . . It seems to me quite possible that all the things that are told to us to-day in analysis as phantasy . . . were once real occurrences in the primaeval times of the human family, and that children in their phantasies are simply filling in the gaps in individual truth with prehistoric truth" (L, 371).

Here is the pinnacle of paradox and the most acute stage of Freud's vacillation. Here is also the ultimate compromise. Freud says: whether neurotics are telling the truth or not is unimportant because even when they are lying they are telling the truth—a prehistoric truth. The fantasies of neurotics are the realities of the primeval human family. The two terms—material reality and psychical reality—initially put forward as being mutually exclusive, are yet at the same time completely inclusive of each other. (Psychical) reality is a fantasy and fantasy is (prehistoric) reality.

The same degree of paradox can be found in Freud's long discussion—in his case study of the Wolf Man, finished in 1914, published in 1917—of the choice between the infantile scenes called primal and a fantasy also called primal. Freud devotes a great number of pages to a minute description of the "primal scene," laboriously attempting to demonstrate the indisputable reality of the child's observation (at the age of eighteen months) of parental intercourse. However, countering his own previous efforts, Freud entertains the possibility that the traumatic primal scene might in fact be a primal fantasy, that is, a universal form of fantasy, independent of personal realities since it is said to derive from the collective prehistoric experiences of the human race. For more detailed information on this question, he refers his readers to the twenty-third of his *Introductory Lectures,* which we have been studying. It is rather difficult, if not impossible, to imagine that the concept of primal fantasy, as expounded in the *Introductory Lectures,* should provide a satisfactory answer to Freud's vacillation about truth and falsehood. Perhaps the most direct formulation of the unresolved dilemma that continued to haunt Freud can be glimpsed in a sentence he added in 1918 to his case study of the Wolf Man: "I intend on this occasion to close the discussion of the reality of the primal scene with a *non liquet*" ("From the History of an Infantile Neurosis," SE 17:60). Is it reality or fantasy? For Freud there is always doubt; it is never quite clear or certain. (We discuss a reemergence of this doubt in Freud between 1929 and 1932 in Part III).

* * *

Judging from the twenty-third chapter of his *Introductory Lectures,* the question of the authenticity of infantile seduction scenes—raised for the first time in September 1897 and apparently resolved right away—in fact was never resolved for Freud. In this continuing vacillation we find the question itself most astonishing as Freud prescribes a choice between reality and fantasy. Analyzing patients with this uncertainty today—are they telling the truth or not?—would amount to adopting Freud's own preoccupation. Having this question in mind would be tantamount to supposing and perhaps even to inducing opposite intentions on the part of patients. In stating that neurotics have little regard for material reality, that they have an unconscious tendency to substitute their fantasies for reality, is Freud attributing to his patients a problem that continually tormented him?

It is questionable whether the analyst's function includes taking a position, making a tacit or explicit judgment about the veracity of the patient's account. Queries concerning reality or invention, truth or falsehood should not arise unless they emerge from the patients themselves. But in this case, we are dealing with a symptom, a behavior to be analyzed and to be situated in its original context. Here are a few situations of this type. A patient surprises us by saying repeatedly over long periods of time, Everything I told you yesterday about the events of my childhood was a lie. It behooves us to analyze the source of this vacillation between truth and falsehood. Who is this patient when she posits the event as real, who is she when she deems it unreal? We need to "accompany" her among her family members, identifying, for example, the person who wants to disguise a shameful event (a suicide, madness, incest, violent crimes, an illegitimate birth, and so on).

In another case, someone is trying to confuse a child by saying, What you thought you saw was only a dream. This patient's hesitation between reality and fantasy aims at re-creating, in the analyst, the sense of bewilderment he himself experienced as a child. Another example: two adults are fighting over a child's trustworthiness as a witness, in the child's presence. One of them is saying, He saw it clearly, he told me so; the other retorts, No, he doesn't understand anything, he is confused, he probably had a nasty dream. In saying to the analyst, Everything I told you yesterday was false, the patient could be referring to the scene in which the adults tried, as it were, to cut him in half. Another case: a father confides a secret about his love life to his young son, asking him not to tell anyone. The subject is never discussed again by the two of them and nobody else talks about it. When this son needs to make his own way in life, asserting himself, saying yes or no, he will flounder and will fall into a pathological form of indecision, to the point of wondering whether what is happening to him right now is just a dream. Yet another situation: the family is attempting to conceal from the child a painful and, if divulged, dangerous reality. But snatches of overheard and suddenly interrupted conversations, evasive and complicitous looks, plant doubt in her heart. The child's questions are met with cold silence or subterfuges meant to throw her off the scent. When grown up, this child will waver until she is dizzy and will never be able to decide whether what she is being told is true or false.

It is dangerous to hold that the distinction between reality and fantasy has no validity in the realm of psychopathology or psychotherapy. We know many a dramatic case in which the analyst's unwillingness to acknowledge the reality of traumatic experiences (emotional devastation of war, deportation, denial of the right to mourn a secret lover, identity crises following incidents of racial or ideological persecution) can lead to profound depression and even madness. In many cases the analyst's function is precisely to bring to the surface a traumatic reality that, because of its painful nature, has dropped from sight, gone underground, and kept silent. It is imperative for analysts to identify the dead areas of one's being—areas sacrificed by the trauma—in order to revive them to the free circulation of speech and life. For those in pain, it is crucial to have people acknowledge the authenticity of their suffering and the reality of the circumstances leading to it.

With no chance to appreciate the full extent of Freud's vacillation between reality and fantasy, most of his disciples have opted for the primacy of fantasy and for a certain distrust of real events. This can result in serious analytical mishaps. The freedom to fantasize is crucial in the formation of the self in childhood and remains an integral part of the harmonious functioning of the adult psyche—this is our conviction. But the problem does not vanish. Imagine a man who speaks in psychotherapy about his sufferings in a concentration camp and who hears from his analyst: Your experiences would have been quite different if, by that time, you had settled your unconscious fantasy of killing your father. (Translated into classical Freudian terms, this means: the neurotic effect of specific incidents on the adult psyche is determined largely by the person's regressions to and fixation at one of the stages of infantile libidinal development.) The potential impact of such a remark on the patient may be difficult to measure for those of us who were schooled in the Freudian doctrine of instinctual fantasies. Yet to mention the unconscious fantasy of patricide, just as the patient is painfully recalling a time when people were preparing to exterminate him—does this not risk plunging him into even greater despair?

II

*Psychoanalysis in the
Eye of Literature*

Applied Psychoanalysis in Question

We reject all attempts to discredit Freud's achievement. Though highly critical, our inquiry issues from an unshakable conviction of the value of psychoanalysis. To cite only the unconscious, infantile sexuality, the psychoanalytic dialogue, the battle against prejudices that would stigmatize mental turmoil—we treasure the liberating thrust of Freud's enterprise. Still, critical vigilance spurs us to question. The questions we put to Freudian psychoanalysis arise from its own inherent methodological paradoxes. We are exploring how and why psychoanalysis in effect counteracts itself, as if behind Freud's luminous genius there lurked a contrary spirit, bent on laying trap after trap. Are dreams stenographic signs whose universal signification is permanent, or do dreams convey the dreamers' singular and personal meaning? Should the interpreter look for innate psychic matter, supposedly common and invariable among all humans, or rather for the constantly shifting mental creations of individuals? These are some of the hesitations, the unresolved questions, if not indeed the genuine theoretical contradictions that seem to us embedded in the Freudian doctrine of dream interpretation. Vacillation and conceptual rifts of this kind occur more than once in Freud's thought. We see the clearest expression of his clinical and theoretical vacillation in the troubled history of infantile seduction—a theory Freud first rejected, then reinstated, abandoned yet again, and in the end amalgamated with the very conception he had proposed as its replacement (see Chapters 1 and 2).

Why should Freud not be contradictory? Was he not the lone and heroic inventor of psychoanalysis? This very fact surely entitles him to having the odd inconsistency overlooked as we hold fast to the indisputable worth of his theories. Yet if Freudian psychoanalysis has major internal contradictions, can it define its own object without controversy? It is necessary to assess the scope and the depth of the contradictions of Freud's thought in all of his works, impartially and in detail. Assailing his tenets in the abstract, without a careful study of the texts, does Freud an injustice and deprives us of the ability to understand the precise nature of his shortcomings. We call for such a comprehensive critical project here, and we initiate it by isolating representative patterns of contradiction in Freud's theories of mental functioning, his study of literature, his clinical practice, and his institutional activities.

Retroactive assessments of Freud's case studies are complicated by the fact that we have only Freud's side of the story; although that reveals a great deal about the originality of his method as well as about his techniques of indoctrination, we will never have a clear picture of the actual dialogue or be able to hear the patient's own voice. A partial remedy is available if we turn to Freud's literary analyses. They are often just as complete as his case studies, and the exchange—or rather the dialogue of the deaf, as the French would call it—can be readily reconstructed since

Freud treats literary characters as if they were patients on his couch. In this chapter we explore how and why Freud's program of applying established psychoanalytic doctrine to literary works collides with his own ambition to shape psychoanalysis into an investigative discipline based on case-specific clinical insights.

Freud's first extended commentary on literature, "Delusions and Dreams in W. Jensen's 'Gradiva'" (1907), is a charming text, bubbling with light-hearted seriousness; it takes its place in the classic series, after Dora (1905) and before little Hans (1909), of Freud's complete psychoanalytic accounts. Leafing through the essay, readers can sense Freud's intention to furnish a veritable manual of psychoanalysis. His theories on dreams, instinctual life, fantasy, and repression—the principal components of his discoveries as of 1907—have a privileged place here. Indeed Freud sees the chief interest of *Gradiva* in its being "a perfectly correct psychiatric study" (DDJ, 43). Consequently, Freud draws a close parallel between Jensen's story (originally published by the Austrian author in 1903) and his own ideas; he offers it as an independent confirmation of his "fundamental theories of medical psychology" (DDJ, 43) in the realm of literature.

Jensen's *Gradiva* provides a mirror of psychoanalysis for Freud, a place where psychoanalysis can come upon its own previously made discoveries, recognize *in vivo* its earlier hypotheses. Freud not only expounds his central theory of sexual repression, he also sees a unique opportunity to discuss his therapeutic procedure through Zoe Bertgang, one of the characters in the tale. On reading his own work, Freud might well have had the impression that *Gradiva* was nothing short of Freudian psychoanalysis, seductively transformed into a fairytale of love. All the requisite elements came together—the patient, his symptoms, dreams, sexual repression—even a psychoanalyst, appearing suddenly as if by magic, to cure the hero in an ideal psychotherapy of love. This is the sweet illusion, Freud's own and that of his willingly enchanted readers—so long as we do not read Jensen's *Gradiva* on its own terms, without Freud's refracting mirror.[1]

Freud's study of *Gradiva* in 1907 marks a significant stage in the evolving scope of psychoanalytic theory. For the first time Freud leaves behind the clinical arena of his research—psychopathologies and their varying manifestations in hysteria, obsessional neurosis, sex life, dreams, and jokes—to establish a continuity between literature and clinical psychoanalysis. From 1907 on the commonality of literature and psychoanalysis furnishes an ever more frequent source of theoretical demonstration. In the *Studies on Hysteria* (1895) Freud wrote that his case studies read like short stories. With *Gradiva* the reverse appeared to him equally plausible: literature exhibits the findings of psychoanalysis. Freud presents his essay on *Gradiva*—published as the first installment of a planned series of monographs, under the general title "Papers on Applied Mental Science"—with a brief programmatic prospectus: "The papers . . . will present in each instance a single study, which will undertake the application of psychological knowledge to subjects in art and literature, in the history of civilizations and religions" ("Prospectus for *Schriften zur angewandten Seelenkunde*" [Prospectus for Studies in Applied Psychoanalysis], SE 9:248).[2]

Throughout his career Freud upheld this program of expanding the range of psychoanalysis in important works such as *Leonardo da Vinci and a Memory of his Childhood* (1910), *Totem and Taboo* (1913), *The Uncanny* (1919), *The Future of an Illusion* (1927), and *Moses and Monotheism* (1939). Though largely concerned with popularizing his discoveries, or perhaps precisely for this reason, the essays on applied psychoanalysis represent those essential aspects of Freud's theory which he wished to communicate to the widest possible audience. For example, he wanted the readers of his commentary on *Gradiva* to understand as a matter of course that sexual repression constitutes the basis of most of our psychological ills and that psychoanalysis has opened a way to undo the repression. Freud sought to introduce sexual repression in this manner as a reliable principle of explanation both in clinical psychotherapies and in the fictive psychotherapy of literary characters.[3] But literary characters on occasion contradict his interpretation and prompt Freud, wittingly or unwittingly, to bend them to the dictates of his theory. The result is that Freud's commentary is quite alien to Jensen's *Gradiva*.[4]

Make no mistake: we salute in Freud the emancipator who opens the hearts and minds of both educators and society to the inmost passions of the child. We pay homage to the advocate who would free us from our own noxious repressions, the enlightener who would tear down all prisons—emotional, sexual, or cultural. We appreciate the extent to which the desire to understand, to resolve everything in the realm of the psyche and beyond, for the sake of humanity and for the well-being of individuals, guided Freud throughout his career and, of course, as he was writing his essay on *Gradiva*. Already in 1905, in his *Three Essays on the Theory of Sexuality,* and even more explicitly in "The Sexual Enlightenment of Children" (published in 1907, concurrently with "Delusions and Dreams in W. Jensen's 'Gradiva'"), Freud admonishes parents and educators to respect the child's questions in matters of sexuality. Trying to put an end to close-minded child-rearing, Freud argues that the thirst for sexual knowledge is naturally inextinguishable in children. He would like to see our society respond to the child's need for enlightenment in sexual matters, and he warns that withholding knowledge may result in pathology because children may remain permanently inhibited in their emotional and intellectual creativity.

In 1907 Freud condemned repressive education, and yet at the same time he limited the free self-expression of literature. We have no quarrel with either the intrinsic value or the therapeutic validity of the theory of sexual repression, an idea that, as Freud has convincingly shown, permits the smooth resolution of countless psychological conflicts. The psychotherapy of sexual repression is an eminently liberating instrument when analysts use it to restore to people the life of desire that has been crushed under the oppressive weight of decades of self-censorship or internalized parental and societal prohibitions. All of Freudian psychoanalysis is based on the discovery of the paramount psychological importance of the vicissitudes of the infantile sexual instinct. The theory of repression also guides Freud's most profound reflections on the relation between the individual and society and on the simultaneously libidinal and repressive origins of civilization itself.

Still, we may be laying a trap for ourselves, for the people we hear in analysis, and for the literary works we cherish, if, because of preconceived ideas, we want them to exhibit forms of pathology from which they do not in fact suffer—regardless of whether the initial discovery of the particular pathology was revolutionary and has since yielded unimpeachable therapeutic results. Freud subjects *Gradiva* to this paradoxical treatment: he forces the literary text before him into the prefabricated mold of dynamic repression. This is typical of Freud's attitude when he urges the use of "applied" psychoanalysis. The application of previously acquired psychoanalytic knowledge is short-sighted because it excludes the possibility of meeting, of welcoming, the new and the unknown. Exporting even the most fruitful psychoanalytic idea outside its proper sphere carries the risk of expunging the singular spirit of individual human beings, literary works, or historical phenomena. In addition, applied psychoanalysis keeps its practitioners from enriching the clinical and theoretical stock of psychoanalysis. (It is important to distinguish here between the application of psychoanalytic doctrine, such as the Oedipus complex, to literature and the unbiased use of psychoanalytic methods of discovery. Thus the Freudian idea that postulates the possibility of gaining insight into unconscious motivation through a given symptomatology allows for complete freedom of interpretation because it merely outlines a discovery procedure and does not prejudge either the content or the structure of the problem at hand.)

We see in the use of applied psychoanalytic doctrine one of the most widely disseminated Freudian paradoxes. We ask the same basic question here as about Freud's contradictory theory of dream interpretation. Should the interpreter rely on an authoritarian code of stable meanings, or instead foster the individual and unforeseeable mental creations of the analysand—even though these personal productions may indeed reach us initially through set expressions, proverbs, myths, legends, stereotypes, or any number of other forms of collective representation? (See our discussion of the expression "old rake" in Chapter 1.) Applied psychoanalysis uses a predetermined conceptual apparatus; it masters the unknown, it subdues the unforeseen through earlier discoveries. Even as it makes use of genuine insights (for example the idea of sexual repression), this kind of psychoanalysis denies literary works the right to speak in their own voice.

A Case Study in Literary Psychoanalysis: Jensen's Gradiva

Many of our readers are familiar with *Gradiva* only from Freud's commentary. Touching and convincing though it may be on its own terms, Freud's reading does not flow from Jensen's tale. To convey the fundamental disparity between Jensen's *Gradiva* and Freud's, we will first juxtapose summaries of Freud's and our own interpretations. (This might turn out to be one of those unfortunate cases of my word against yours, were it not that (1) *Gradiva* is available for all to read and judge and (2) it is relatively easy to trace the paths of distortion Freud uses to bend the story to his predetermined conception.) Next, in a more extended literary psychoanalysis, we will attempt to restore *Gradiva* to its own distinctiveness and to show that it is possible to illuminate literature through psychoanalysis, provided that the text is not used as a handmaiden of theory. Following our account of the story we will analyze the paradoxes and distortions that result from Freud's forcible application of sexual repression in a context where this idea has no place, no reason to be.[5]

• • •

In Freud's version *Gradiva* tells of Norbert Hanold, a young German archaeologist who lives in total isolation, devoting himself exclusively to his professional interest in Greco-Roman Antiquity. One day he acquires the plaster cast of an ancient bas-relief. After fabricating an imaginary world for the woman represented on the relief, the archaeologist begins studying the gait of contemporary women. He compares them to their ancient counterpart on the plaster specimen (to which he gives the name Gradiva) and finally discovers someone on the street who seems to correspond quite exactly to the relief. Thereupon, "without realizing that he was acting under the influence of delusion" (as Freud puts it), he suddenly flees his home, leaving for Italy and ending up in Pompeii. His unconscious flight from the beloved woman (actually a childhood friend) is due to the repression of his sexuality:

> His childhood friendship, instead of being strengthened into a passion, was dissolved, and his memories of it passed into . . . profound forgetfulness. (DDJ, 34)

> Norbert Hanold's memories of his childhood relations with the girl . . . were repressed . . . The ancient relief aroused the slumbering erotism in him, and made his childhood memories active. On account of a resistance to erotism . . . , these memories could only become operative as unconscious ones. What now took place in him was a struggle between the power of erotism and that of the forces that were repressing it; the manifestation of this struggle was a delusion. (DDJ, 48–49)

It is the delusion of being in love with the sculpture of a woman and later with her ghost. In Pompeii Norbert believes he has found the ghost of Gradiva. According to Freud, Jensen situates his story in Pompeii to show that Norbert Hanold unconsciously equates his repressed childhood with the burial of Pompeii:

"There is, in fact, no better analogy for repression . . . than burial of the sort to which Pompeii fell a victim . . . Thus it was that the young archaeologist was obliged in his phantasy to transport to Pompeii the original of the relief which reminded him of the object of his youthful love" (DDJ, 40). Norbert arranges to meet the ghost several times. At the end of their fourth meeting, he and a young woman leave the ruins of Pompeii hand in hand, having decided to get married. This is the upshot, according to Freud, of a cure performed by Zoe Bertgang, alias Gradiva, the long-forgotten friend from Norbert's childhood. "The procedure which the author makes his Zoe adopt for curing her childhood friend's delusion shows a far-reaching—no, a complete agreement in its essence—with a therapeutic method which was introduced into medical practice in 1895 by Dr. Josef Breuer and myself, and to the perfecting of which I have since devoted myself" (DDJ, 88–89).

Here now is the gist of our analysis of Jensen's *Gradiva*. The young archaeologist Norbert Hanold pursues a family tradition of classical scholarship. Quite abruptly he loses both his parents. In an unwittingly endured illness of mourning, he comes to identify with them as deceased. For years Norbert lives as if dead, prizing only inanimate objects and the remnants of extinct civilizations. One day he buys the ancient relief of a young woman, shown in an energetic stride, and this marks the beginning of the end of his emotional coma. His fancies and daydreams based on this effigy, and the idea that it memorializes someone named Gradiva who really perished in 79 A.D., lend an indirect voice to his silent grief. Though unaware of the link to his own situation, Norbert engages with the fictitious Gradiva in all the characteristic acts of the survivor who, dejected at first, grows resigned to the loss. Witnessing Gradiva's death in a nightmare, he buries her, so to speak, yearns over her, and cherishes the bas-relief as her monument. With this soothing release of grief, Norbert embarks quite unknowingly on an ever more impassioned search for life and love. He travels to Pompeii and there invents Gradiva's miraculous return as a ghost, thus staging, as though in a dream, his incredulous joy at discovering his own revival. Jensen's choice of Pompeii therefore does not indicate an analogy with the process of sexual repression as Freud has argued. Rather, as a site of cataclysmic destruction, Pompeii embodies the hero's principal symptom, namely the pain of sorrow that for a time has made life repellent to him. His "cure" ensues without anybody's intervention quite simply because in time life triumphs over the devastation of death. For years Norbert has been stuck in stone like Gradiva; then he is resurrected in the very house of death, in Pompeii, and marries Zoe, his rediscovered love of life.

Freud's interpretation of *Gradiva* says: Norbert Hanold's sexual repression censored the infantile object of love (Zoe), and created the delusion of his archaeological fantasy about a woman cast in stone (Gradiva). Thus Norbert fled the unconsciously loved real woman; in his flight he chose Pompeii because the erstwhile burial of this city resembled his own psychic process of sexual repression. Though untrained, Zoe turned out to be a successful analyst because her private feelings for Norbert led her to adopt quite readily the ultimate aim of psychoanalysis, the restoration of the capacity to love.

There would be few reasons to question Freud's commentary if it did not refer to an autonomous literary work. But *Gradiva* does not corroborate his interpretation. The story contains absolutely no sexual repression, no flight from the beloved, no psychoanalyst, and no justification for Freud's analogy between dynamic sexual repression and the burial of Pompeii.

Dear reader, allow us to present in some detail the psychoanalytic unfolding of Jensen's story. We take you on this emotional journey because we want to share with you our heartfelt and seasoned conviction that psychoanalysis can offer a unique avenue for understanding human beings and their creations, provided that we can identify and shake off those aspects of the Freudian method which endanger the freedom of psychological investigation.

In our eyes Jensen's *Gradiva: A Pompeian Fancy* (1903) provides a modern-day version of the ancient Pygmalion myth. Pygmalion, the king of Cyprus, fell in love with the statue of a woman. Seized with passion, he begged Venus to give him a woman in the statue's likeness. Shortly thereafter the statue came to life, and he went on to marry her. Jensen tells of a young archaeologist who falls in love with the statue of a maiden; she later comes to life in Pompeii under his gaze. Her real name is Zoe, "life" in Greek. The archaeologist confesses his love to her and proposes marriage.

Jensen uses central elements of the Pygmalion myth, enriching it with a new psychological dimension. In the ancient version of the myth, Ovid had already assigned a reason for Pygmalion's unusual passion. Shocked at the vices nature bestowed on women, Pygmalion lived celibate and gave his statue a beauty beyond what nature could grant. Jensen invents a different explanation for his hero's celibacy and his love for a lifeless statue: the trauma of mourning. Through this psychological motivation Jensen deepens the original myth. It is no longer the statue that comes to life through Venus's intercession but the grief-stricken young man; from being emotionally dead, he is transformed into a lover of life. In Ovid's *Metamorphoses* the myth takes only a couple of pages to tell. Jensen's version is much longer and rather more indirect because it depicts a largely unwitting, internal transformation in which the passage of time and the succession of events play major roles. At first the hero is surprised to find passions in himself, and only very gradually does he realize the true nature of his feeling for the statue and its alleged reincarnation. He gives the statue a name, imagines for her a life and a death in the ancient city of Pompeii; he conceives the desire to see her live again; when he later meets her in Pompeii, he is overwhelmed by doubts as to whether she is a ghost or a flesh-and-blood creature; bit by bit he settles his doubts and unravels all the extravagant notions that were merely tokens of his as yet fragile attachment to life.

Our analysis of *Gradiva* will occur in three parts: (1) the hero's sinuous path to his own sexuality; (2) his emotional death and gradual revival; and (3) his unconscious grief, the cause of his temporary withdrawal from life.

The Rousing of Vital Desire in Norbert Hanold

"The thought that others might also speak to her, . . . made him indignant. To that he alone possessed a claim . . .; for he had discovered Gradiva . . ., had observed her daily, taken her into his life and, to a degree, imparted to her his life-strength, and . . . thereby again lent to her life that she would not have possessed without him" (G, 209).

This outburst of jealous love—for Gradiva, a fictive being, followed immediately by a declaration of love to Zoe, a real woman—encapsulates the hero's progress by the end of Jensen's tale. It is a slow progress, made of dreams, fantasies, apparently bordering on delusion but in reality constantly accompanied by flashes of insight. Norbert Hanold starts on his emotional journey right after discovering the Roman relief of a young woman. He wraps the marble creature in a magical circle of thoughts; he invents Greek origins for her and fantasizes about her daily existence near Mount Vesuvius just prior to its eruption and the destruction of Pompeii.

"So the young woman was fascinating . . . chiefly by the movement represented in the picture . . . This movement produced a double impression of exceptional agility and of confident composure" (G, 148). Why does Norbert fill his head with a woman of stone? To place in her subtly evolving image his own unconsciously budding desires. He calls his emotional creation Gradiva, "the girl splendid in walking" (G, 148). Movement will be the paradoxical essence of a woman immobilized in stone because she symbolizes the progress Norbert is about to make. Arrested in his emotional advance as if he were himself a marble figure, Norbert admires the statue's gracefully resolute step forward. "Gradiva, 'the girl splendid in walking.' That was an epithet applied by the ancient poets solely to Mars Gradivus, the war-god going out to battle" (G, 148–149). Though as yet unaware, Norbert derives the name Gradiva from Gradivus because he sets out to conquer a woman who, with Gradiva's splendid step, might hasten to meet him as well.

In the mirror-like reflection between the relief and Norbert, Gradiva and her fascinating walk indicate the gradual stirring of a desire to love and be loved. In the next episode Norbert throws himself headlong into finding this ideal manner of walking among the women of his native town. "His desire for knowledge transported him into a scientific passion in which he surrendered himself to the peculiar investigation . . . Among all, however, not a single one presented to view Gradiva's manner of walking" (G, 152–153). Are Norbert's observations quite fruitless? Not at all, since they mark a decisive internal movement forward. For Norbert "women had formerly been . . . only a conception in marble and bronze, and he had never given his female contemporaries the least consideration" (G, 152). Heretofore utterly indifferent, he now makes the female sex the object of an impassioned quest:

> Then something like a thrill passed through him; in the first moment he could not say whence . . . Down in the street, . . . a female . . . was walking along with easy, elastic step . . . Quickly Norbert Hanold was in the street without

> knowing exactly how he had come there. He had . . . flown
> like lightning down the steps, and was running down among
> the carriages, carts, and people . . . His glance was seeking
> the young lady."   (G, 156–157)

For a moment "he thought he had seen not the face of a stranger but that of Gradiva looking down upon him" (G, 158).

Gradiva is all around Norbert now. More than a relief on his wall, she is a constant longing in his daydreams, the coveted object of his examination of the gait of women, a fleeting apparition on the streets of his home town. The first stage of Norbert Hanold's nascent desire culminates here; it is a desire that has developed little by little over the years, in his solitary companionship with the statue of Gradiva.

The unexpected rush of feeling unsettles the reclusive life of the orderly young archaeologist, bent above all on enhancing the brilliant family tradition of learning and classical scholarship. Yet, with Gradiva's all-consuming presence about him, a vague sense of captivity awakens in him. Norbert feels caged like the bird across the way. "Thus Norbert Hanold . . . was thereupon moved by the feeling that he, too, lacked a nameless something" (G, 160). Does Norbert yearn for a flesh-and-blood Gradiva? Unable to realize this, he comforts himself with the thought that he is quite unlike the caged canary because he has wings, if only he wants to use them; and he definitely will now. Soon after Gradiva's flit across the street, he decides impulsively to take a spring trip to Italy. He "cast at nightfall another regretful departing glance on Gradiva" (G, 160). To discover the life of his desire—Norbert senses this obscurely—he must forever quit the marble Gradiva.

Before finding a real Gradiva, Norbert will take in many sights—more internal than external perhaps; he shuttles between oppressive feelings of captivity and bouts of passionate desire in a dead city. A site of death and a site of love, Pompeii is from here on the scene of Norbert's twofold itinerary, leading him toward emotional freedom and the discovery of love. Meanwhile the unknown intensities of his emotion shock him. The flies in Pompeii drive him into a seething rage. "He had never been subject to violent emotions; yet a hatred of these two-winged creatures burned within him" (G, 170). Norbert is no longer in control. His outbursts as yet waver—taking shape variously as loathing of flies or contempt at smooching honeymooners—but his nascent passions all but take over. In Rome, where he travels "to inform himself about some important archaeological questions in connection with some statues" (G, 161), "a strangely oppressive feeling had again taken possession of him, a feeling that he was imprisoned in a cage which this time was called Rome" (G, 165). Norbert's sense of dissatisfaction grows in Pompeii: "Pompeii, too, apparently offered no peacefully gratifying abode for his needs. To this idea was added another, at least dimly—that his dissatisfaction was probably not caused by his surroundings alone, but to a degree had its origin in him . . . He felt that he was out of sorts because he lacked something without being able to explain what" (G, 171–172).

The sensation of an inner lack overflows all of Norbert's thoughts and emotions to the point of rendering him utterly indifferent to archaeology. A nameless rousing abruptly transforms Pompeii, the most precious of archaeological sites, into a rubbish heap of useless knowledge: "Not only had all his science left him, but it had left him without the desire to regain it; he remembered it . . . old, dried-up . . ., the dullest and most superfluous creature in the world . . . What it taught was a lifeless, archaeological view, . . . a dead, philological language. These helped in no way to a comprehension with soul, mind, and heart, or whatever one wanted to call it" (G, 179). Dismissing archaeology, the initial pretext of his trip to Italy, Norbert is now ready to encounter the object of his yearning. At that precise moment, as if conjured by passionate enchantment, Gradiva "stepped forth . . . buoyantly . . . Here, however, it was not in a stone representation . . . As soon as he caught sight of her . . . he became conscious of something else; he had, without himself knowing the motive in his heart come to Italy . . . and had without stop, continued . . . to Pompeii to see if he could here find trace of her" (G, 180–181).

Haunted thereafter by the living mirage of Gradiva, Norbert will use her image to complete his emotional journey. Seizing as well on various small incidents of his life as a tourist in Pompeii, he will recognize the twofold and interconnected reality of the young woman before him and of his love for her. Notwithstanding his initial hesitation as to Gradiva's reality, he never doubts the vital renewal she has produced in him: "Had what had just stood before him been a product of his imagination or a reality? . . . Yet he felt from the secret inner vibrations that Pompeii had begun to live about him . . ., and so Gradiva lived again, too" (G, 182).

Who is living again here, Pompeii, Gradiva, or Norbert? Jensen provides the answer in the second half of his story. The encounter with a young woman gives shape to Norbert's desires, a desire for life and love, conceived and nurtured earlier in his shared existence with the statue of Gradiva: "He had found what he was looking for, what had driven him unconsciously to Pompeii; Gradiva continued her visible existence in the noonday spirit hour and sat before him" (G, 186). Is it mere chance or rather Jensen's mischief that supplies at this precise stage the real name of Norbert's sentimental cares? The name is Zoe, "life" in Greek. In a subtle mixture of kindhearted warmth and benevolent irony, Jensen puts before our eyes, one by one, the unfolding blossoms of Norbert's growing love of life.[6]

Norbert's overexcited imagination is now on fire. Insignificant events, such as the sight of a pair of lovers kissing or the purchase of a metal brooch, will act as catalysts. A series of unforeseen incidents (which include the meetings with Zoe Bertgang) quickens the pace of Norbert's internal advance toward openly wanting to love a living woman. He gradually allows the outside world to seep into him, ultimately shaking off the wild fictions of his mind. Meanwhile a merchant cheats Norbert into buying a brooch that allegedly belonged to a Pompeian couple "who had clasped each other in fierce embrace when they realized their inevitable destruction and had thus awaited death" (G, 205). Norbert convinces himself that the brooch was Gradiva's. Thus he discovers that intimacy can exist between Gradiva and a man. He also repeatedly observes a young couple of tourists. Thinking at first that they are brother and sister, Norbert knows better when he sees them locked in a passionate kiss. This pair of lovers impresses him. Through them he realizes his growing passion for Zoe-Gradiva. About to meet her, he prepares to grapple with an imaginary rival:

> When he arrived before the house of Meleager . . . he was equally afraid of not meeting Gradiva within, and of finding her there; . . . in the first case, she would be . . . somewhere else with some . . . man, and, in the second case, the latter would be in company with her . . . Toward the man, however, he felt a hate . . .; until today he had not considered it possible that he could be capable of such violent inner excitement. The duel, which he had always considered stupid nonsense, suddenly appeared to him in a different light . . . So he . . . stepped forward to enter; he would challenge the bold man. (G, 212–213)

Having wanted Gradiva all to himself, Norbert tells her of his joy at seeing her still alive, at being with her. "'I believed at first that you could be here only during the noon hour, but it has become probable to me that you also, at some other time—That makes me very happy'—'Why does it make you happy?' . . . Confused, he offered, 'It is beautiful to be alive; it has never seemed so . . . to me before'" (G, 214–215). His heart now open, Norbert longs to clarify the physical nature of his companion. He has little doubt any more that she is a flesh-and-blood creature, but Gradiva's confusing jests force him to make an experiment:

> So, for a little while, the couple did not speak further . . . until Gradiva said, "It seems to me as if we had eaten our bread like this once, two thousand years ago. Can't you remember it?" He could not, but it seemed strange to him . . . The idea that she had been going around here in Pompeii such a long time ago would no longer harmonize with sound reason; everything about her seemed in the present, [she] could be scarcely more than twenty years old.
>
> (G, 216)

Norbert will strike his partner's hand as a fly sits on it and will know whether it is a real, living hand or not. The unmistakably warm bodily contact will confirm his intuition.

Another unexpected event prompts Norbert to lay aside forever the already inoperative figments of his imagination, the fictions that had situated Gradiva at the center of the destruction of Pompeii. Directly after the incident of the fly on Gradiva's hand, the couple he has watched kissing appear. "At the same time there sounded in the colonnade footsteps . . .; before his confused eyes appeared the faces of the congenial pair of lovers. . ., and the young lady cried . . ., 'Zoe! you here, too? And also on your honeymoon?' . . . Norbert was again outside . . . How he had come there was not clear to him; it must have happened instinctively" (G, 218).

Norbert is suddenly overcome with shame. He wants to avoid appearing ludicrous in the eyes of the people whose friendship and love he so ardently desires: "Of course it seemed . . . unquestionable that he had been utterly foolish and irrational to believe that he had sat with a young Pompeian girl, who had become more or less corporeally alive again" (G, 223). Nothing at all stands in his way now. His wild notions melt away, and Zoe—who delights in teasing him about his long neglect of their former friendship—can hear from the young man himself the token of his emotional liberation: "What luck, though, that you are not Gradiva, but are like the congenial young lady!" (G, 230). Tasting the joys of love, Norbert bursts out lyrically, "Zoe, you dear life and lovely present—we shall take our wedding trip to Italy and Pompeii" (G, 234). The Gradiva of his solitary dreams fades and makes way for the exhilaration of life, Zoe, the rapture of love.

It is clear now: where Freud saw a struggle with sexual repression, Jensen's story showed a path to love.

Norbert Hanold's Death and Revival

Norbert's gradual recognition of his erotic desires moves through multiple levels of reality. Starting from an unconscious infatuation with a young woman made of stone, he progressively turns toward himself; his emotions stun him. Hitherto unknown wishes, bouts of anger, impulsive acts overtake him; the stirrings of the soul and the body signal a want to the young man. His emotional crisis climaxes when he meets "Gradiva" amid the ruins of Pompeii, when he thinks he sees the noontide ghost of a woman he supposes died nearly two thousand years earlier. While no more than a bundle of fantasies reaches the surface—the former existence in ancient Pompeii of a young woman later cast in stone, her ghostly return amid the contemporary ruins of Pompeii, her death in the arms of her lover, and now the miracle that she again possesses a body—this sequence of seemingly wild fictions outlines definite stages in the emergence of Norbert Hanold's maturing desire. As adolescents wake up to their bodies, suddenly recognize their sexual needs, and long for romantic encounters,

Norbert too builds a constantly shifting structure of imagination about the other sex.

But Norbert Hanold, a well-respected archaeologist, is no longer an adolescent. Why then the delay in his erotic development? Other questions arise as well. Why does Norbert's sexual awakening attract him—in his fancy, in his dreams, and in the form of an actual trip—to Pompeii, a dead city? Why does he build his daydreams for years around the stone image of an allegedly Pompeian woman? Why does he believe he has met the ghost of a person who had died in a cataclysm some two thousand years before? In short, why does the young man's sexual rousing rely on the imagery of death? This still requires an explanation.

It is appropriate to speak of a delayed maturation of erotic desire in Norbert's case—but not of its repression. The distinction is crucial. No Freudian repression whatsoever exists in Jensen's tale, because there is no opposition or compromise between two contrary psychic trends. The protagonist's daydreams and insights show instead his unstoppable progress toward the open embrace of his nascent sexuality.

Freud states that Jensen "omitted to give the reasons which led to the repression of the erotic life of his hero" (DDJ, 49). However, Jensen's story is unconcerned with sexual repression, and the psychological reasons for the hero's behavior stand out if, following the text, we understand this: Jensen's creature suffers from a temporary death of desire as the consequence of a traumatic loss. Freud imposes on the story the notion of a battle between opposing psychic forces. Norbert is not the scene of an insidious struggle between sexual drives and their censorship. He is the unsuspecting victim of a disaster that has nearly extinguished his zest for life. The premature death of his parents has led to an *illness of mourning* in Norbert. The grief over the loss of his family merged with a hidden sorrow of his heart, body, and soul as their incipient awakening was abruptly stifled.[7]

Throwing the reader *in medias res* into the thick of Norbert's private fantasies, Jensen later clarifies the young archaeologist's family situation and present condition. We see in this passage the crucial elements that help explain the psychological source of Norbert's behavior, including both his love of a stone creature and his peculiar Pompeian fictions:

> From his early childhood no doubt had existed in his parents' house that he, as the only son of a university professor [of classics], was called upon to preserve . . . that very activity . . . He had clung loyally to it even after the early deaths of his parents had left him absolutely alone; in connection with his brilliantly passed examination in philology, he had taken the prescribed student trip to Italy . . . Nothing more instructive for him than the collections of Florence, Rome, Naples . . . That, besides these objects from the distant past, the present still existed round him, he felt only in the most shadowy way; for his feelings marble and bronze were not dead, but rather the only really vital thing . . .; and so he sat in the midst of his walls, books, and pictures, with no need of any other intercourse, but whenever possible avoiding the latter . . . and only very reluctantly submitting to an inevitable party, attendance at which was required by the connections handed down from his parents. Yet it was known that at such gatherings he was present without eyes or ears for his surroundings, . . . and on the street he greeted none of those whom he had sat with at the table.

(G, 158–159)

During his adolescence Norbert Hanold prematurely lost both of his parents. His profession is no doubt the legacy of a family tradition, but, given his present circumstances, it has taken on an additional function. Archaeology allows him to pursue unconscious contact with the dead through the study of past civilizations that like his family were once vibrant and are now extinct.

Jensen's story follows Norbert's recovery from the emotional and sexual anesthesia inflicted by death. He, who for a time had all but stopped living, gradually returns to life, finding it incarnate in a person endowed with a poetically significant name: Zoe Gradiva Bertgang—life that, with a splendid walk, steps forward.

Unlike Freud, we do not think that Zoe Bertgang undertakes anything even remotely resembling psychotherapy. She does indeed press Norbert with questions about his odd fantasies. She does so, however, with the sole purpose of testing whether it is possible to rekindle her former companion's interest in her. Zoe teases Norbert, mocking him shamelessly: "Don't you recall having eaten together like this two thousand years ago?" She wants to learn about Norbert's quaint fondness for the ghost of a long-dead Pompeian because she believes she can substitute her flesh-and-blood self for the imaginary woman. This is why she offers herself in unambiguous terms as the genuine object of desire for her now estranged but once close friend. When the young man is clearly ready to shed his cocoon of isolation, she tells him of their lost friendship, their adolescent pranks, Norbert's incomprehensible withdrawal later on, and the total lack of contact between them since then.

Zoe offers no explanation for his behavior. If she considers anyone from a psychoanalytic point of view, it is not her friend but herself. She understands fully the reason for her enduring attachment to Norbert in the face of his utter indifference. Having lost her mother early on, Zoe had practically no father either as he always cared more for zoology than for her. Norbert's affection and joyful presence had brought a ray of sunshine into her empty family life. Even after this faithful and cheerful companion had almost irretrievably vanished, Zoe continued to cherish her long-time friend from childhood and adolescence. She hoped that friendship might someday change into a feeling of shared love, the fulfillment of her adult life. In her speech Zoe provides Norbert with this lucid insight into her own psychology.[8] She would undoubtedly have refrained from laying bare her thoughts unless she felt implicitly invited to do so, unless she could see that Norbert had freed himself sufficiently from his extravagant dream world and could now view her as she really was. Still, given her psychological sagacity, it is quite possible that she might one day want to find out why Norbert withdrew so radically from life and why he entertained such peculiar Pompeian fantasies—but this, the hero's tender and loving psychoanalysis by Zoe, is not in the story Jensen wrote.[9]

Norbert Hanold's Grief and Fantasies of Pompeii

Norbert Hanold's revival borrows the imagery of Pompeii's destruction because of the abrupt loss he suffered and the lengthy illness of mourning that resulted from it. Had his been a case of uncomplicated erotic awakening, Norbert could have derived some feminine image from a real person or the aspirations and experiences he shared with his teenage friends. When no obstacle exists, the libido of adolescents adapts to the progressive shifts of self-asserting desire and defines itself through contact with real people. But Norbert chose a woman of stone on an ancient and inanimate relief. Her life had allegedly been spent in Pompeii, a city doomed to destruction. Norbert's daydreaming exhibits all the qualities of adolescent love fantasies save for one thing: the images rising up before him relate to the effigy of someone whose irrevocable death he witnessed in a nightmare:

> He had, one night, a dream which caused him great anguish of mind. In it he was in old Pompeii, and on the twenty fourth of August of the year 79 A.D., which witnessed the terrible eruption of Vesuvius . . . All the inhabitants . . . stunned out of their senses . . ., sought safety in flight. The pebbles and the rain of ashes fell down on Norbert also, but

. . . they did not hurt him . . . As he stood thus at the edge
of the Forum . . ., he suddenly saw Gradiva a short distance
in front of him . . . So with buoyant composure and the
calm . . . peculiar to her, she walked across the flagstones
. . . She seemed not to notice the impending fate of the city
. . . Then, however, he became suddenly aware that if she
did not quickly save herself, she must perish in the general
destruction, and a violent fear forced from him a cry . . . At
the same time, her face became paler as if it were changing
into white marble; she stepped up to the portico of the
Temple, and then, between the pillars, she sat down on a
step and slowly laid her head upon it. Now the pebbles were
. . . condensed into a completely opaque curtain; hastening
quickly after her . . ., he found the place . . ., and there she
lay . . . as if for sleep, but no longer breathing, apparently
stifled by the sulfur fumes. From Vesuvius the red glow
flared over her countenance, which, with closed eyes, was
exactly like that of a beautiful statue.   (G, 153–154)

The nightmare of the eruption of Mount Vesuvius is so posi-
tioned in Jensen's tale that, on reading the hero's poignant biography four pages later, the reader should be able to make a natural
connection between Gradiva's imagined passing and the real
death of Norbert's parents. Is it surprising then that Norbert is
devoted to archaeology, that he takes refuge in the study of
fragments rescued from dead civilizations? "That, besides these
objects from the distant past, the present still existed round him,
he felt in the most shadowy way; for his feelings marble and
bronze were not dead, but rather the only really vital thing"
(G, 159).

The lifeless relief of a dead person is an appropriate token for
the painful reality of someone ill from mourning: "When Norbert
Hanold awoke, he still heard the confused cries of the Pompeians

who were seeking safety . . . With woeful feeling he now viewed . . . the old relief, which had assumed new significance for him. It was, in a way, a tombstone by which the artist had preserved for posterity the likeness of the girl who had so early departed this life" (G, 155). If Norbert convinces himself that the stony Gradiva of his dream memorializes a premature Pompeian death, it is because this thought gives him an indirect opportunity to grieve over the loss of his loved ones and to weep over his own bereavement. Seeing Gradiva die so young in Pompeii amounts to seeing his youthful hopes dashed by the shock of untimely death. Norbert's fantasies about Pompeii and the petrified life of Gradiva have their source in the traumatic reality of his own abruptly stifled vital desire.

His fantasies relative to revival, Gradiva's ghostly visitation and Pompeii's rebirth, tell of his unwitting attempts to recover life after the disaster of death. Thus the stone Gradiva spontaneously vanishes into thin air as soon as life definitively triumphs in Norbert. His fantasies are quite simply replaced by the love growing up between two young people, Norbert Hanold and Zoe Bertgang.

The statue of Gradiva and her imaginary "half-life" in Pompeii mirror the stages of Norbert's victory over his illness of mourning. In the transitional state of mourning—in which nothing is truly alive or dead—the reemergence of vital desire depends on the degree to which the pain inflicted by death can subside. Hence the twofold and complementary nature of Norbert's imaginary creation. Gradiva captures the simultaneously evolving internal processes that resolve grief and usher in the rebirth of desire. Having dreamed of Gradiva's death, Norbert leaves for Pompeii to find some trace of her. Norbert's emotional progress now hinges on the reality and duration of Gradiva's revival. The day after first meeting the "ghost" Norbert is desperate, thinking he will not find Gradiva at the appointed hour and place. Does

Gradiva only live "in the noon hour of spirits" (G, 194)? Questions like these torment him. It was true only "the day before, perhaps the one time in a century or a thousand years, for it suddenly seemed certain that his return today was in vain. He would not meet the girl he was looking for, because she was not allowed to come again until a time when he too would have been dead for many years, and would be buried and forgotten" (G, 194). Translation: Norbert has not yet fully recovered from the life-sapping effects of bereavement. It is hard for him to believe in a lasting revival, much less in a definitive one.

The uncertainty draws from him a spontaneous expression of hunger for life as he notices Zoe: "Oh, that you were still alive!" (G, 194). Oh, that I were alive, Norbert tells himself, using the image of Gradiva since he cannot as yet formulate this wish with respect to himself. In his hand he is holding an asphodel, the flower of the underworld, that he will give to the Gradiva of his still-doubting self. Are the faint signs of vital renewal mere deception? The uncertainty makes Gradiva's real name seem inappropriate: "'I didn't know your real name and don't know it yet' . . . 'My name is Zoe' . . . With pained tone the words escaped him: 'The name suits you beautifully, but it sounds to me like bitter mockery, for "Zoe" means life'" (G, 199). For Norbert life is but mockery, and at best a passing dream. For years he has lived like the dead, like someone for whom only occasional and fleeting returns to life are permitted. He is like Gradiva's supposed ghost that walks, with the grave flower at the noon hour, along the lava blocks, near the Street of Tombs in Pompeii. Can a ghost, an entity forever hovering between life and death, have a body? This question now overtakes Norbert even as he thrills to hitherto unknown emotions: "What was the nature of the physical manifestation of a being like Gradiva, dead and alive at the same time?" (G, 194). The question he raises in terms of Gradiva of course pertains to Norbert himself.

"His knowledge of medicine was not comprehensive . . . , but this strange condition must arise from excessive congestion of the blood in his head, perhaps associated with accelerated action of the heart; for he felt the latter—something formerly quite unknown to him—beating fast against his chest. Otherwise, his thoughts . . . continually turned about the question of what physical nature Zoe-Gradiva might possess" (G, 202). Norbert's questions about his body by way of Gradiva's intensify through chance meetings. To the question—Am I alive?—others are added. Can I have physical desires, be in love, clasp my beloved and receive her love in return? Norbert asks all these questions indirectly by reflecting on Zoe-Gradiva's nature or her supposed possessions and activities. For example, he strains his wits over a brooch that "burned his fingers as if it had become glowing" (G, 206). Did this brooch, allegedly found near the remains of a couple locked in embrace at the time of Pompeii's destruction, belong to Gradiva?

Whatever the answer, Norbert profits because his thoughts about the pair of Pompeian lovers bring him ever closer to the direct expression of his own desire for life and love. Soon Norbert will be able to love and even demand exclusive reciprocity from his lover. "The thought that others might also speak to her, . . . made him indignant. To that he alone possessed a claim . . . ; for he had discovered Gradiva, had observed her daily, taken her into his life and to a degree, imparted to her his life-strength, and . . . thereby again lent to her life that she would not have possessed without him" (G, 209). He still requires the reciprocity of feeling from Gradiva, his own living-dead imaginary creation. The hour is near, however, when he will want the exclusive love of a living woman, for example someone similar to Gisa Hartleben, a person he met by chance. He observes this friend of Zoe's just as he sets out to meet his own Gradiva. The scene of the kiss transforms his fantasy of the perished Pompeian couple into a living image: "His eyes clung to the living picture, more widely open than they had ever been to any of the most admired works of art . . . [he] ran out with bated breath and beating heart" (G, 212).

Little by little life pushes back the shadows of death in Norbert. He thinks now that Gradiva's life can extend beyond the noon hour. At their next meeting he replaces the asphodel with the rose; he gives her the flower of passion, not the white symbol of the realm of death: "Her hand stretched out to receive the red flowers, and, handing them to her, he rejoined, 'I believed at first that you could be here only during the noon hour, but it has become probable to me that you also, at some other time—That makes me very happy . . . It is beautiful to be alive; it has never seemed so . . . to me before'" (G, 214–215). Life asserting itself ever more, Norbert willingly leaves behind the somber cloud land of fantasy he has invented. "Of course it seemed . . . unquestionable that . . . Gradiva was only a dead bas-relief" (G, 223).

Norbert's emotional progress from the lifeless limbo of grief to vibrant erotic maturity replaces the statue of the dead Gradiva with a living woman. Life, the name of his future wife, Zoe, encapsulates the psychological road Norbert has traveled. In Zoe Bertgang he reclaims the ardor of life.

The Distortions of Psychoanalysis:
Freud versus Jensen

Why is it important to consider in detail the disparities between Freud's commentary on a literary work, such as Jensen's *Gradiva,* and the work itself? Freud repeated throughout his career that his clinical work formed the bedrock of his entire psychoanalytic edifice. His unprejudiced understanding of individual cases and his therapeutic success with patients constituted both the impetus and the incontrovertible empirical evidence for his psychological theories. Yet, as our look at his fictive case study of Jensen's *Gradiva* shows, Freud actually hindered the progress of his own discipline by adopting self-defeating methodologies. At one and the same time, his methods opened and closed the doors of psychological comprehension. Freud achieved highly original insights to make psychological sense of emotional ills, but he also chained these very insights to clinical or literary cases that failed to corroborate them. Even as he vowed unheard-of openmindedness in dealing with individual psychological pain, he forced previously gained clinical knowl-

edge onto people and texts with vastly different kinds of pathologies from the ones to which that knowledge applied.

In the same way, Freud often distorted his own unique procedures of discovery by constraining them in predetermined directions. For example (and we will say more of this later in this
chapter), he showed conclusively in *The Interpretation of Dreams*
that to understand senseless or disjointed dreams it was necessary
to assume various forms of distortion or disguise, such as the
combination of the actions of two or more separate people into
a single person. Yet, while Freud insisted that such distortions and
disguises could be grasped and removed only with the aid of the
dreamers' own commentary on their dreams, he often laid down
a catalog of stable and universally applicable rules for distortion,
such as that anxiety in dreams must always stand for sexual excitement. Freud's own desire to force his cases into his preconceived theoretical models has insidiously undermined the effectiveness of psychoanalysis as a whole.

Freud and Pompeii: Repression or Death?

Freud's account of *Gradiva* describes a severely pathological case
of sexual repression that manifests itself in delusions and necessi-
tates another person's intervention for its cure. Jensen's story
portrays the spontaneous progress of emotional and sexual rebirth in a young man trapped for years by an illness of mourning
but now eager for life and love.

Freud's need to fit *Gradiva* into his model of sexual repression
at all costs led him to the conjunction of two incompatible ideas:
(1) the protagonist suffers from sexual repression; (2) the mechanism of sexual repression in him resembles the fate of ancient
Pompeii.

(1) Norbert Hanold's erotic feelings . . . were repressed;
and since his erotism knew and had known no other object

than Zoe Bertgang in his childhood, his memories of her were forgotten . . . What now took place in him was a struggle between the power of erotism and that of the forces that were repressing it; the manifestation of this struggle was a delusion. (DDJ, 49)

(2) There is, in fact, no better analogy for repression, by which something in the mind is at once made inaccessible and preserved, than burial of the sort to which Pompeii fell a victim and from which it could emerge once more through the work of spades . . . The author [Jensen] was well justified, indeed, in lingering over the valuable similarity which his delicate sense had perceived. (DDJ, 40)

We see the opposite: no connection exists between the dynamic repression of a person's love life and the burial of Pompeii either in Jensen's *Gradiva* or in Freud's own theory of repression. The incongruity looms large in 1907 and intensifies in Freud's so-called papers on metapsychology from 1915, namely "The Unconscious" and "Repression."

Freud, the inventor of the concept in the realm of psychopathology, defined repression as a conflict, the incessant struggle between two contrary psychical tendencies, censorship and the return of the repressed (the content of which is said to be most often erotic in nature). Repression concerns the latent or unconscious states of mental life and is used by Freud to describe a mechanism that rejects them. The aim of repression is to suppress or inhibit an erotic "instinctual impulse from being turned into a manifestation" that would be directly available to consciousness (U, 178–179). However, the repressed impulse keeps fighting its way back toward consciousness with the help of substitutive representations and disguised images. The conflict endures because, even as repression works to remove the rejected impulse from consciousness, "the repressed idea remains capable of action in the Ucs [Unconscious]" (U, 180). Given two opposing forces—the inextinguishable energy of the repressed and the equally persistent pressure of repression—the unconscious attachment to the rejected erotic idea either is "discharged in the form of anxiety" or takes "flight" in substitutive ideas "by displacement" (U, 182). In the neurotic symptom the repressed erotic impulse is displayed but only in the distorted form allowed by repression.

It is important to note that Freud presented these very precise views on repression extensively for the first time in his essay on *Gradiva:*

> "Repressed" is a dynamic expression, which takes account of the interplay of mental forces; it implies that there is a force present which is seeking to bring about all kinds of psychical effects . . . but that there is also an opposing force which is able to obstruct some of these psychical effects.
>
> (DDJ, 48)

> The symptoms of a delusion—phantasies and actions alike—are in fact the products of compromise between the two mental currents, and in a compromise account is taken of the demands of each of the two parties to it; but each side must also renounce a part of what it wanted to achieve. Where a compromise comes about it must have been preceded by a struggle—in this case it was the conflict we have assumed between suppressed erotism and the forces that were keeping it in repression. In the formation of a delusion this struggle is in fact unending. Assault and resistance are renewed after the construction of each compromise.
>
> (DDJ, 52)

Can Pompeii, its destruction, and its burial fit into these descriptions? A constant mental force, repression repulses active unconscious impulses that nevertheless unceasingly reappear in disguise, insidiously borrowing their masks from the very materials employed against them by repression. Is it really this perennial conflict between the instinctual impulse and its repression that Freud likens to the burial of Pompeii? Paradoxically, yes. However, "the valuable similarity" seems mysterious if not outright incomprehensible in light of Freud's own statements. He writes in 1907: "We can assert quite definitely of 'repression' that it does not coincide with the dissolution or extinction of the memory" (DDJ, 34). He is even more explicit in "The Unconscious" in 1915: "We have learnt from psycho-analysis that the essence of the process of repression lies, not in putting an end to, in annihilating, the idea which represents an instinct, but in preventing it from becoming conscious" (U, 166). The essay "Repression" strengthens this view: "The process of repression is not to be regarded as an event which takes place *once*, the results of which are permanent, as when some living thing has been killed and from that time onward is dead" (R, 151).

Of the two alternatives, only one is viable. Was Pompeii annihilated once and for all in 79 A.D., to be from that time onward dead? Or has Pompeii, in its buried existence, continued to be dynamic, capable of rearing its head like repressed mental acts, and ready to produce at any time insidiously distorted, latent effects? The answer seems obvious, and yet Freud says: "There is, in fact, no better analogy for repression . . . than burial of the sort to which Pompeii fell a victim" (DDJ, 40). How to resolve such a clear-cut contradiction? Can we imagine Pompeii after its destruction in terms of unceasing activity as the Freudian theory of repression would require? "Repression demands a persistent expenditure of force, and if this were to cease the success of the repression would be jeopardized, so that a fresh act of repression would be necessary" (R, 151). Can Pompeii's annihilation and burial be made to parallel the struggle between an erotic impulse and its repression? "We may suppose that the repressed [impulse] exercises a continuous pressure in the direction of the conscious, so that this pressure must be balanced by an unceasing counter-pressure. Thus the maintenance of a repression involves an uninterrupted expenditure of force" (R, 151).

The gap between the Freudian theory of dynamic repression and the image of Pompeii is unbridgeable. Freud's essay from 1907 and his subsequent writings from 1915 effectively preclude the comparison. Worse yet, they suggest that the destruction of Pompeii is in fact the perfect counterexample of dynamic repression. Had Freud proposed Pompeii merely as an expedient analogy, who would feel compelled to scrutinize its cogency? However, he wanted to persuade his readers that no better analogy exists for repression, and he anchored his interpretation of *Gradiva* on this flawed analogy. We must raise the question then with respect to Jensen's *Gradiva:* Is ancient Pompeii the best analogy for the Freudian idea of repressed unconscious drives or, instead, the image of instantaneous, catastrophic, irrevocable death—and mourning?

Jensen and Pompeii: A Freudian Blind Spot

Freud mentions *Gradiva* once more, somewhat disparagingly, in 1924 in *An Autobiographical Study,* but without altering his initial interpretation: "I was able to show from a short story by W. Jensen called *Gradiva,* which has no particular merit in itself, that invented dreams can be interpreted in the same way as real ones and that the unconscious mechanisms familiar to us in the 'dream-work' are thus also operative in the processes of imaginative writing." (SE 20: 65). Of course we know that Freud wrote his essay "Mourning and Melancholia" (1915) eight years after his commentary on *Gradiva.* Let us dream for a moment. Our psychoanalysis of Jensen's hero—the progressive resolution of his illness of mourning, his belated arousal to life and love—could have occurred in Freudian terms, if Freud had broadened his definition of the *work of mourning,* an idea he introduced in 1915 in "Mourning and Melancholia." However, this is creating a pious fiction, since no text by Freud indicates any intention on his part to change his original interpretation. "Delusions and Dreams in W. Jensen's 'Gradiva'" has remained paradigmatic of dynamic sexual repression and of the role Pompeii was to play as an exemplary image of this type of repression. The fictive future of Jensen's *Gradiva* in the potential development of Freudian theory is not the focus of our inquiry. We want to evaluate Freud's actual interpretation from 1907—with respect to which he never varied—in the face of the story by Jensen.[10] Following a brief summary of our results so far, we will analyze in detail the techniques of distortion (as concerns the role of Pompeii in particular) Freud used to bend the story to his preconception.

Freud's commentary merely appears to treat Jensen's *Gradiva.* In reality, Freud leaves out or deforms its essential characteristics: he neglects the link between the idea of Pompeii's destruction and the hero's grief. He pushes aside the text's fundamental questions, all of which concern death and the potential recovery of life. Why is the hero attracted in his dreams, imagination, and travel to Pompeii, a city destroyed in a volcanic cataclysm? Why does the ancient sculpted likeness of a woman call up in Norbert Hanold images of Pompeii's destruction? Once in Pompeii on an impulsively arranged trip, why does he believe the city is suddenly reviving? Why does he think that a young female visitor to the excavated city is actually the ghost of one of the victims who perished there in 79 A.D.? Why does he want to see her return to life? Disregarding the twofold subject of the story, grief and revival, Freud's approach obeys a series of foregone conclusions: the writer, like the psychiatrist, is interested in pathological mental states; I have discovered the repression of instinctual life; this is an absolutely essential perspective in the explanation of psycho-pathological phenomena (compare DDJ, 43–45 and 53–54); Jensen fictionalizes mental pathology, therefore he draws on the issue of sexual repression (DDJ, 54).

Freud has diagnosed a conflict supposedly giving rise to delusions that might have become fixed if not for some form of therapeutic intervention. The psychotherapy Freud attributes to Zoe thus grows out of his preconception of sexual repression and the treatment that would be necessary to relieve its delirious symptoms. With this notion of an ideal love-cure performed by Zoe, Freud casts aside Norbert's fully autonomous progress in Jensen's story: the young man evolves along two parallel tracks, resolving his grief even as he ripens his desire for romantic union.

Norbert's development shows in his autonomous shift from Gradiva to Zoe, from the sculpture of a dead person to a vital and desirable woman. The hero's visions, imaginations, and hallucinatory fantasies concerning Gradiva give metaphorical shape to his internal evolution. Even his most fantastic conceits are no more than transitional expressions of a gradual alteration in his inner realities; all his extravagant notions fade one by one because they are not meant to last; each is a step overtaken by the next and ultimately discarded as soon as grief yields to the attraction of life. The two figures, Zoe and Gradiva, need to be viewed as the external marks of an emotional process within Norbert. The inanimate relief, the dream of Pompeii's destruction, the trip to Pompeii, the encounter with Gradiva's ghost, and finally Zoe provide the means to show Norbert's illness of mourning and his emotional revival, his mute despair and his renewed desire for life. Jensen's tale uses apparently unrelated events, objects, and people to display the changes the hero cannot identify in himself.

Freud tells us that Norbert flees to Pompeii. "His journey was a result of his resistance gathering new strength . . . ; it was an attempt at flight from the physical presence of the girl he loved.

In a practical sense it meant a victory for repression" (DDJ, 67). However, the story rejects Freud's interpretation. There is neither repression nor a return of the repressed. Norbert's trip means a victory for life as his dejection lifts. In Pompeii he stops being a lifeless marble statue; he looks for Gradiva's living trace and turns toward life with the idea that the dead can revive.

The hero has to get over a catastrophe—the tragedy of grief— so he can live again. This evolution, taking him from the anesthesia of sorrow to the revival of life, has nothing to do with repression, a struggle between two mutually exclusive mental tendencies. By introducing repression and the conflicting return of the repressed, Freud blocks out the substance of Jensen's text: the irretrievable destruction of Pompeii, the very metaphor that indicates the extinction of life in Norbert Hanold.

If we examine the commentary, we see that Pompeii poses a major interpretive problem for Freud. Jensen's story bears the subtitle *A Pompeian Fancy,* but Freud's analysis transforms it into an *archaeological* fancy. Whereas the fundamental psychological fact of Jensen's story is the hero's preoccupation with Pompeii, Freud bases his analysis on eroticism's being disguised behind an interest in archaeology. "The interest taken by the hero of the story in this relief [of Gradiva] is the basic psychological fact in the narrative" (DDJ, 11). This premise does not include the idea of Pompeii as a dead city. Even as he sees in *Gradiva* "a case history and the history of a cure which might have been designed to emphasize certain fundamental theories of medical psychology" (DDJ, 43), Freud disputes the relevance of Pompeii in several key episodes of the story. The meeting between Norbert and Zoe in Pompeii is one of these "premises which do not seem to have their roots in the laws of reality" (DDJ, 41); the writer "makes the young man meet the living woman precisely in Pompeii" where "the dead woman had been placed . . . only by his imagination" (DDJ, 42). For Freud this meeting in Pompeii derives from "chance, which unquestionably plays a part in many human histories" (DDJ, 42). He later concludes: "Apart from this, it must be repeated, the author has presented us with a perfectly correct psychiatric study, on which we may measure our understanding of the workings of the mind" (DDJ, 43). It is therefore only by omitting Pompeii and by replacing it with archaeology that Freud can say, "for a number of years . . . I myself have supported all the views that I have here extracted from Jensen's *Gradiva*"(DDJ, 53). Freud thus feels able to describe Norbert Hanold's presumed psychopathology fully without any need to question the psychological import of Pompeii's overwhelming presence in Hanold's imagination.[11]

Here are the major components of Freud's analysis:

Archeology took hold of him and left him with an interest only in women of marble and bronze. His childhood friendship, instead of being strengthened into a passion, was dissolved, and his memories of it passed into such profound forgetfulness that he did not recognize or notice his early playmate when he met her in society . . . There is a kind of forgetting which is characterized by the difficulty with which the memory is awakened . . ., as though some internal resistance was struggling against its revival. A forgetting of this kind has been given the name "repression" in psychopathology; and the case which our author has put before us seems to be an example of this repression . . . What is repressed cannot, it is true, as a rule make its way into memory without more ado; but . . . under the influence of some external event, it may one day bring about psychical consequences which can be regarded as products of a modification of the forgotten memory . . . We have already seemed to recognize in Norbert Hanold's phantasies about Gradiva derivatives of his repressed memories of his childhood friendship with Zoe Bertgang . . . If Norbert Hanold were someone in real life who had in this way banished love and his childhood friendship with the help of archeology, it would have been logical and according to rule that what revived in him the forgotten memory of the girl he had loved in his childhood should be precisely an antique sculpture. It would have been his well-deserved fate to fall in love with the marble portrait of Gradiva, behind which . . . the living Zoe whom he had neglected made her influence felt.

(DDJ, 34–37)

Freud here gives his complete assessment of Norbert Hanold's pathology, but the fate of ancient Pompeii does not figure in it. The idea of Pompeii emerges after the analysis is over. However, the initial omission and subsequent adjunction of Pompeii are hardly noticeable in Freud's text. The reader is dazzled as Pompeii, absent until then, suddenly seems to spring up everywhere:

(1) The author has presented us with a key to the symbolism of which the hero's delusion made use in disguising his repressed memory. There is, in fact, no better analogy for repression, by which something in the mind is at once made inaccessible and preserved, than burial of the sort to which Pompeii fell a victim and from which it could emerge once more through the work of spades. Thus it was that the young archeologist was obliged in his phantasy to transport the original of the relief which reminded him of the object of his youthful love. The author was well justified, indeed, in lingering over the valuable similarity which his delicate sense had perceived between a particular mental process in the individual and an isolated historical event in the history of mankind. (DDJ, 40)

(2) Once he had made his childhood coincide with the classical past (which it was so easy for him to do), there was

a perfect similarity between the burial of Pompeii . . . and repression, of which he possessed a knowledge through what might be described as "endopsychic" perception.

(DDJ, 51)

(3) In her conversations with Hanold . . . Zoe [is] using the same symbolism that we found in Hanold's first dream—the equation of repression and burials and of Pompeii and childhood.   (DDJ, 84–85)

In this he was using the same symbolism that the author makes the girl use consciously towards the conclusion of the story.   (DDJ, 51)

Did Freud remove Pompeii entirely from his psychoanalysis of Norbert? No matter, since retroactively he makes Pompeii overspread the interpretation.

For Freud's readers Pompeii now provides an analogy raised to the second power, a metapsychological allegory of mental processes that are in themselves quite devoid of the idea of Pompeii. Freud tantalizes us and himself with the opportunity to see in the fate of ancient Pompeii a privileged image of his own theory of dynamic repression. The Pompeian analogy of repression must have appealed to Freud as it allowed him to liken a significant event in the early history of mankind to the laws of individual depth psychology. This type of comparison—for example between the beliefs of so-called primitive peoples and the psychological makeup of contemporary neurotics—became one of the hallmarks of Freud's style as he sought ever more striking confirmation of his tenets.

Yes, the similarity between dynamic repression and Pompeii can achieve a synthesis—somewhat belatedly since it occurs after Freud has completed the analysis of sexual repression in Jensen's hero, but a synthesis nonetheless and one that loses none of its metaphorical allure. The analogy between repression and the burial of Pompeii does at first sight appear quite irresistible. Is it not highly plausible that an archaeologist should seize on Pompeii "because no other or better analogy could be found in his science for his remarkable state, in which he became aware of his memories of his childhood through obscure channels of information" (DDJ, 51)? It might seem no less reasonable to see in Pompeii and its excavation an echo of the psychoanalytic work that, according to Freud, Zoe performs.

Will the characters, the author, and the readers of the story surrender, one by one, to Freud's charm? The hero's imagination supposedly carries him to Pompeii because he unconsciously divines the Freudian analogy between the burial of Pompeii and his own sexual repression. In the same way, Zoe psychoanalyzes him almost as Freud might. Finally, Jensen calls his work *A Pompeian Fancy* because his "delicate sense had perceived" better than anybody else "the valuable similarity" Freud established "between a particular mental process in the individual and an isolated event in the history of mankind" (DDJ, 40). Freud fascinates us all, and his spell ends up bewitching him as well. He wonders whether Jensen did not in fact base his fiction directly on Freudian theories.[12]

Yet beyond this charm Freud's analysis Freud strips Pompeii of its characteristics in the context of Jensen's *Gradiva:* death, destruction, and grief. Freud pushes aside the disaster of death both in tying dynamic repression to Pompeii and in his analysis of Norbert Hanold's psychological motivation. In two crucial instances Freud omits—wittingly or unwittingly—a reference to grief, even though Jensen indicates it clearly. The first omission occurs in the brief biography of Norbert Hanold, a passage in which Jensen explains Norbert's isolation through the premature death of his parents. Juxtaposing the relevant quotations from Freud and Jensen, we see that Freud transcribes everything but one detail. Here is Freud:

Our hero's . . . behavior . . . still appears to us as incomprehensible and foolish . . . It is the author's privilege to be allowed to leave us in such uncertainty. The charm of his language and the ingenuity of his ideas offer us provisional reward for the reliance we place in him and . . . his hero. Of this hero we are further told that he was preordained by family tradition to become an archeologist, that in his later isolation and independence he was wholly absorbed in his studies and had turned completely away from life and its pleasures. Marble and bronze alone were truly alive for him.

(DDJ, 14)

And here is Jensen:

From his early childhood no doubt had existed in his parents' house that he, as the only son of a university professor [of classics], was called upon to preserve . . . that very activity . . . He had clung loyally to it even after the early deaths of his parents had left him absolutely alone . . . Nothing more instructive for him than the collections of Florence, Rome, Naples could be offered anywhere . . . That, besides these objects from a distant past, the present still existed round him, he felt in the most shadowy way; for his feelings marble and bronze were not dead, but rather the only really vital thing. (G, 158–159)

A piece of information about Norbert's parents—"the early deaths of his parents had left him absolutely alone"—does not appear in Freud's summary; therewith disappears the direct link between the hero's recent loss and his refusal to live in the present.

Another instance of Freud's deletion of grief occurs in his interpretation of Norbert's main dream. The manner of the exclusion here is quite different. Freud's summary of Jensen's text scrupulously reproduces the idea of Pompeii's destruction—but the commentary removes it. Behind Pompeii's devastation and Norbert's grief Freud wants to see the distorted features of an entirely disparate set of latent thoughts. This is Freud's transcription of Jensen's text.

> He had a terrifying dream, in which he found himself in ancient Pompeii on the day of the eruption of Vesuvius and witnessed the city's destruction . . . he suddenly saw Gradiva at no great distance from him. . . When he hurried after her, he found her stretched out on the broad step with a peaceful expression, like someone asleep, till the rain of ashes buried her form. When he awoke . . . he retained his belief for a long time in the reality of what he had dreamt . . . The dream had as its result that now for the first time in his phantasies about Gradiva he mourned for her as someone who was lost. (DDJ, 12–13)

Here now are the most significant parts of Freud's lengthy analysis of the dream in which he transforms the expression of mourning into a disguised representative of latent erotic thoughts:

> Thus interpreting a dream consists in translating the manifest content of the dream into the latent dream-thoughts, in undoing the distortion which the dream-thoughts have had to submit to from the censorship of the resistance. If we apply these notions to the dream we are concerned with, we shall find that its latent dream-thoughts can only have been: "the girl you are looking for with the graceful gait is really living in this town with you." But in that form the thought could not become conscious. It was obstructed by the fact that a fantasy had laid it down . . . that Gradiva was a Pompeian; consequently . . . there was no other choice

but to adopt the distortion: "You are living in Pompeii at the time of Gradiva." (DDJ, 59)

The sense is merely disguised in a particular way so that it is not immediately recognizable. Hanold learned in the dream that the girl he was looking for was living in a town contemporaneously with him. Now this was true of Zoe Bertgang; only in the dream the town was not the German university town but Pompeii, and the time was not the present but the year 79 A.D. It is, as it were, a distortion by displacement; what we have is not Gradiva in the present but the dreamer transported into the past . . . But whence come this displacement and disguise which were bound to deceive both us and the dreamer over the true meaning and content of the dream? . . . Now let us suppose that dream-images are . . . the creations of people's . . . delusions—the products of the compromise in the struggle between what is repressed and what is dominant [in the conscious personality] . . . We shall then understand that dream-images have to be regarded as something distorted, behind which something else must be looked for, something *not* distorted.

(DDJ, 58–59)

Are we perhaps under an obligation to replace in this way each separate piece of the manifest content of the dream by unconscious thoughts? Strictly speaking, yes. (DDJ, 60)

For Hanold's dream was an anxiety-dream. Its content was frightening, the dreamer felt anxiety while he slept and he was left with painful feelings afterwards . . . The anxiety in anxiety-dreams, like neurotic anxiety in general, corresponds to a sexual affect, a libidinal feeling, and arises out of the libido by the process of repression. When we interpret a dream, therefore, we must replace anxiety by sexual excitement. . . On that basis, we should say that the dreamer's erotic longings were stirred up during the night . . . but that those longings met with a fresh repudiation and were transformed into anxiety, which in its turn introduced into the content of the dream the terrifying pictures from the memories of his schooldays. In this manner the true unconscious content of the dream, his passionate longing for the Zoe he had once known, became transformed into its manifest content of the destruction of Pompeii and the loss of Gradiva.

(DDJ, 60–61)

In Norbert Hanold's first dream two wishes competed with each other . . . The first was a wish, understandable in any archaeologist, to have been present as an eyewitness at the catastrophe in the year 79 A.D. . . . The other wish, the other constructor of the dream, was of an erotic nature: . . . a wish to be there when the girl he loved lay down to sleep. This was the wish the rejection of which caused the dream to become an anxiety-dream. (DDJ, 93)

In his dream interpretation Freud disputes the veracity of the dreamer's anguish, though Jensen links it directly to the inevitable and catastrophic death of a loved one. Norbert "was in old Pompeii, and the twenty fourth of August of the year 79 A.D., which witnessed the terrible eruption of Vesuvius . . . She [Gradiva] seemed not to notice the impending fate of the city . . . Then, however, he became suddenly aware that if she did not quickly save herself, she must perish in the general destruction, and a violent fear forced from him a cry of warning" (G, 153–154). It is in this anxiety that Freud discerns the distortion of unacknowledged sexual arousal. He claims that Pompeii's annihilation and Gradiva's death effectively mask repressed erotic desires. In support of the dream's latent eroticism he invokes a man's natural desire to be at the beloved girl's side as she lies down to sleep.

Freud's arguments simply annul the text of the dream. For him the beloved lies down to sleep; in Jensen's tale Gradiva lies down stifled—to die. In the story Pompeii's and Gradiva's demise directly raise the question of grief—why does Norbert weep over the relief of a young woman he never met?—yet Freud produces a legion of intricate disguises to show the insidious return of repudiated sexuality.

The dream's interpretation encapsulates the disparity between Jensen's text and Freud's analysis of it. The story sketches a gradual awakening to life and love after the coma of mourning; Freud diagnoses the conflicting and delusional work of sexual repression. Jensen uses Pompeii as the metaphorical stage on which to display the calamity of a life nearly torn asunder by grief; Freud attempts to justify the presence of Pompeii through a complex relation between dynamic repression on the one hand and the burial and excavation of Pompeii on the other. The nightmare of death and destruction in Pompeii fits with logical ease into Jensen's *Gradiva*—no distortion or displacement is needed to grasp its sense. Freud introduces them in order to identify features of his own theory. Having discarded the issue of grief that matters to the hero, Freud feels compelled to neutralize and translate nearly every single detail in his dream.

This is why psychoanalysis with predetermined insights is totally counterproductive: the genuine substance of a text is replaced by an alien entity. The psychoanalytic concepts under application require interpreters to view the intrinsic elements of a text as so many disguises of a preprogrammed meaning they intend to find. The person or the text endures merely as a fictitious entity now defined by the interpreter. Jensen's *Gradiva* has been eclipsed by Freud's.

Despite our sharp criticism of Freud's techniques of distortion, we want to affirm the intrinsic potential of literary psychoanalysis.

We envision literature as a resource for psychoanalytic inquiry, as an enhancement of our growing comprehension of people and their imaginative riches. Like human beings themselves, literary works are forever unforeseeable, and in their uniqueness they offer myriad avenues for expanding our ways and means to understand them. In the exchange between literature and psychoanalytic theory, all privilege must accrue to the text. Encounters between the creative work and the psychoanalyst should lead to theoretical recasting, expansion, or refinement—never to compliance. Instead of rigidly applying its tenets, psychoanalysis must continually adapt to literature. If psychoanalysis is incapable of this openness and flexibility, it may lose its reason for being. Because turning a deaf ear to literature is the same as refusing to embrace the singular essence of each and every human being.

III

Transmissions of Psychoanalysis

Censorship and Secrets in the Historical Topography of Psychoanalysis

All scientific disciplines have their histories, the history of the formation and dissemination of their theories. The history of a set of problems is generally separated from the nature of the problems themselves. Thus the axioms of a given discipline are tested by empirical observation but are not usually challenged by historical examination. For example, no account of the mystical sources of Kepler's cosmology or of the nearly idolatrous reception of Newtonian physics in eighteenth-century France will do anything to damage or enhance the theory's objective validity. Nevertheless, we argue here that the interrelatedness of history and theory is a specific feature of Freudian psychoanalysis. This gives rise to two parallel questions. Does the history of the psychoanalytic movement reveal theoretical contradictions in Freud's work? Or conversely, have the unrecognized internal paradoxes of Freudian theory led to contradictory practices in the institutional transmission of psychoanalysis?

The cohesion of professional Freudianism has been due in great measure to the particular mode of its transmission. Indeed, it is the institutionally monitored personal psychoanalysis of all future analysts that sustains the movement inaugurated by Freud nearly a century ago. In the vast majority of psychoanalytic institutions, candidates are expected to recognize in themselves the psychic structures consecrated by the Freudian legacy—the Oedipus complex, castration, penis envy, the death drive, and so on. Once their personal psychoanalysis is over, future analysts undertake a second, so-called supervised training analysis on the same doctrinal basis. That is, they now seek in their own patients the mental structures they previously identified in themselves. The training analysis, then, generally upholds the basic tenets of Freudian psychoanalysis. The certification of candidates by the International Psychoanalytic Association gives the crowning touch to this process of continued allegiance to the Freudian canon.

Undergoing individual and/or training analysis is arguably the best preparation possible for the professional psychotherapeutic treatment of others. However, this sort of training may perpetuate flaws. And the gravest flaw in this domain is undoubtedly the difficulty of assessing freely the preconditions of one's own adherence to Freud's thought and of reflecting on the peculiarities in the historical transmission of his theories. In a word, the pressures exerted by a mode of teaching that privileges loyalty to the inventor's doctrine hardly encourage, and may even stifle, independent thought and creativity on the part of future practitioners.

Freeing psychoanalysis from its own institutional barriers is not a matter of individual will. Such emancipation cannot occur without investigation of the causes of internal blockage. For this purpose it is useful to envision the institutional transmission of Freudian theories as part of a *historical topography* of psychoanalysis. This historical topography encompasses the life and works of

Freud, of course, but also reaches beyond them to include the activities of the entire psychoanalytic movement, such as the statutes governing psychoanalytic associations, the procedures for selecting candidates, the work of Freud's disciples and biographers, and the writings of the institutional historians, interpreters, and disseminators of his thought.

The history of psychoanalysis is comparable to a vast mental organization that includes, among other features, areas of silence, secrets, and crypts. Wardens of silence rear their heads when we approach Freud's letters. Even though their publication has been under way for over half a century—it was initiated in the 1930s by Marie Bonaparte's acquisition of the Freud-Fliess letters—their release to the public is not complete to this day. For many years the correspondence with Fliess and the letters exchanged between Freud and Ferenczi either were not published at all or were issued in incomplete and expurgated editions. Certainly, Freud's letters have played a major role in the scholarly assessment of psychoanalysis. It is a well-known fact, for example, that Ernest Jones, Freud's authorized biographer, created his version of Freud based on numerous letters the Freud family or its friends placed at his exclusive disposal. In his biography (published between 1953 and 1957) Jones lets us know that he is familiar with letters and documents that, for the most part, have remained out of the public's reach. Thanks to this access to documents and letters, Jones, among the "happy few," commands a privileged view of psychoanalysis and demands from his readers unconditional confidence in the authority of his role as ambassador. But occasional protests have arisen ever since the 1950s over the lack of access to the primary materials of the history of psychoanalysis. The German author Ludwig Marcuse, an intellectual biographer of Freud, wrote to Jones on 10 October 1957 about the Freud-Fliess correspondence:

It is incomprehensible to me why Freud's major correspondence is not being made available to the public in its entirety so that those who would draw Freud's picture should not be limited to expurgated selections. You will most certainly understand that some people, despite their veneration of your book on Freud, wish to see all the materials . . . the desire to arrive at an independent opinion is quite great, at least as far as I am concerned.

(M, 148–149; our own translation)

Now that, thanks to Jeffrey Masson, *The Complete Letters of Sigmund Freud to Wilhelm Fliess* have been published, Jones's attitude, as expressed to Marcuse on 14 September 1957, is puzzling:

You are entirely mistaken in supposing that the family employed me as a censor or that I myself suppressed any material. They gave me carte blanche with the result that reviewers have praised me for the extreme frankness with which I dealt with Freud's intimate life. Where you find data missing in the book you may be sure that they do not exist. Thus I know nothing about the sexual aspect of Freud's marriage and never felt like inquiring from his wife about the frequency of their sexual intercourse. The same applies to the publication of the Fliess correspondence. I have of course read all the unpublished letters. In a few cases I found a couple of sentences of sufficient interest to be worth publishing and Anna Freud promptly did so in the English translation. The rest were entirely uninteresting talks about the weather of a holiday, each other's children, and the date of his resuming work. (M, 144–145)

The "couple of sentences of sufficient interest to be worth publishing" have swollen to over a hundred letters—omitted in their entirety from the original edition of 1950. The claimed triviality of the omitted passages is refuted in a letter Anna Freud wrote to Jones himself on 19 November 1953. This letter provides a spontaneous commentary on the subsequent exchange between Jones and Marcuse: "Emma Eckstein was an early patient of my father's and there are many letters concerning her in the Fliess correspondence which were left out, since the story would have been incomplete and rather bewildering to the reader" (quoted in AT, 55).

Why is censorship—a key concept in Freud's metapsychology and a correlative to the concepts of repression and superego—being applied to the primary materials of psychoanalysis? The reader of Freud's letters is met with a wall of silence within the fortified ego of psychoanalysis. Such is Marcuse's lot, told by Jones to read his biography and called a neurotic along the way, no doubt so that he should give up wanting to ferret out unpublished letters:

> Unfortunately, in writing about Freud's personality in the first chapter [of your book] you have suffered the same fate of the many other approaches to the subject. It seems always to stir some unconscious conflicts which lead to serious misinterpretations and incorrect hypotheses which only add to the distorted legends of that personality which are so frequent. It even affects the capacity to quote correctly simple facts even when they are perfectly clear in my Biography. (M, 145)

What will be the reaction of the Freud scholar? Will Marcuse submit to censorship, recoiling from independent thought and inquiry? Or is there a way for him to examine the role that censorship has played in the history of psychoanalysis? In Jones's letter to Marcuse one can sense a censor's credo: first, my being a censor is itself a secret ("You are entirely mistaken in supposing that the family employed me as a censor"); second, as to what I do conceal, whatever is missing does not exist ("When you find data missing . . . you may be sure that they do not exist"), or, alternatively, what does exist is trivial ("The rest were entirely uninteresting talks about the weather").

There is nothing to be discovered in the unpublished portions of the Freud-Fliess letters. Apart from the potentially embarrassing revelations about Eckstein's operation (Freud's letters tell of his distress after the unfortunate surgery by Fliess on Eckstein's nose), does this statement by Jones cover up an intention to hide Freud's hesitations about the causes of hysteria? Several fragments omitted from the correspondence seem to bear this out. Two examples will suffice here. We should recall that, according to the standard historical interpretation, Freud abandoned his theory of infantile sexual seduction in a letter to Fliess dated 21 September 1897. Yet from another letter, written on 12 December 1897, the following fragment was omitted: "My confidence in the paternal etiology has risen greatly. [Emma] Eckstein deliberately treated her patient in such a manner as not to give her the slightest hint of what would emerge from the unconscious and in the process obtained from her, among other things, the identical scenes with the father" (CL, 286).

In another letter, dated 22 December 1897, a lengthy account of abuse by a father had to be restored:

The intrinsic authenticity of infantile trauma is borne out by the following little incident which the patient claims to have observed as a three-year-old child. She goes into a dark room where her mother is carrying on [sorting out her feelings] and eavesdrops. She has good reasons for identifying herself with this mother. The father belongs to the category of *men who stab women* [deflowerers] for whom bloody injuries are an erotic need. When she was two years old, he brutally deflowered her and infected her with his gonorrhea, as a consequence of which she became ill and her life was endangered by the loss of blood and vaginitis. The mother now stands in the room and shouts: "Rotten criminal, what do you want from me? I will have no part of that. Just whom do you think you have in front of you?" Then she tears the clothes from her body with one hand, while with the other hand she presses them against it, which creates a very peculiar impression. Then she stares at a certain spot in the room, her face contorted by rage, covers her genitals with one hand and pushes something away with the other. The she raises both hands, claws at the air and bites it. Shouting and cursing, she bends over far backward, again covers her genitals with her hand, whereupon she falls over forward, so that her head almost touches the floor; finally, she quietly falls over backward onto the floor. Afterward she wrings her hands, sits down in a corner, and with her features distorted with pain she weeps.

For the child the most conspicuous phase is when the mother, standing up, is bent over forward. She sees that the mother keeps her toes strongly turned *inward!*

When the girl was six to seven months (!!) old, her mother was lying in bed, bleeding nearly to death from an injury inflicted by the father. At the age of sixteen years she again saw her mother bleeding from the uterus (carcinoma), which brought on the beginning of her neurosis. The latter breaks out a year later when she hears about a hemorrhoid operation. Can one doubt that the father forces the mother to submit to anal intercourse? Can one not recognize in the mother's attack the separate phases of this assault: first the attempt to get at her from the front; then pressing her down from the back and penetrating between her legs, which forced her to turn her feet inward. Finally, how does the patient know that in attacks one usually enacts both persons (*self*-injury, *self*-murder), as occurred here in that the woman tears off her clothes with one hand, like the assailant, and with the other holds onto them, as she herself did at the time?

A new motto: "What has been done to you, you poor child?"

Enough of my smut.

(CL, 289; our emendations appear in brackets)

However whimsical the editorial omission of these fragments may seem, they are certainly not devoid of reason. In both cases, references to sexual traumas occasioned by violent fathers are omitted. The editors omitted Freud's statement of renewed confidence in the etiology of infantile seduction in the letter of 12 December 1897—barely two months after his renunciation of it in September. As for the letter of 22 December, the full description of a clinical case was omitted. This case of abuse by a father reinforced Freud's confidence to the point of inspiring a new motto—also deleted—for his research into childhood traumas. (The motto—"What has been done to you, you poor child?"—comes from Mignon's song in Goethe's *Wilhelm Meister.* In the novel, Mignon is an abused child.)

Why, one might ask, obscure by censorship the ups and downs of Freud's thoughts on the etiology of hysteria? Who could fail to see in the series of restored fragments—Emma Eckstein's authenticating discoveries, the case of sexual violence, and the new motto—anything but a revival of the forsaken seduction theory? Ernst Kris and the editorial team of *The Origins of Psychoanalysis: Letters to Wilhelm Fliess* (1954) would probably respond by saying that they did so to safeguard the theoretical coherence of Freud's legacy. After all, in September 1897 he did emphatically reject the reality of sexual violence upon children. To confuse the reader with the master's hesitations would have been counterproductive since his doubts would ultimately seem transitory and slight when compared to the vast system, psychoanalysis properly speaking, that was to follow the "turning point" in September. The editors of the correspondence thus assumed unilaterally the task of protecting a Freudian doctrine they wanted to hand down as unshaken. Yet, as we survey the many vicissitudes of Freud's long-standing vacillation concerning reality and fantasy, it becomes clear that a fundamental upset of doctrinal psychoanalysis was continually haunting Freud himself.

In Freud's letter to Fliess, dated 22 December 1897 and fallen prey to editorial censorship in 1950, a comparison has nonetheless been left intact between the senseless speech of delirium and a text rendered unintelligible by censorship: "Have you ever seen a foreign newspaper which has passed Russian censorship at the frontier? Words, whole clauses and sentences are blacked out so that the rest becomes unintelligible. A *Russian censorship* of that kind comes about in psychoses and produces the apparently meaningless *deliria*" (CL, 289). Circulating Freud's letters with bits happening to pass through such "Russian censorship" has thrown readers and psychoanalysis as a whole into a form of historical neurosis. Because the deletions of primary material have made the open transmission of psychoanalysis very nearly impossible, the institutional constraints of psychoanalysis—at times going so far as to conceal the documents that recount the circumstances of its invention—have taken on symptomatic proportions. As a result the teaching of psychoanalysis has threatened to become unyielding and more often than not has been accompanied by historical omissions, silences, secrets, and purges.

Who took on the role of censor in the historical topography of psychoanalysis? The events leading to the "formation of a *secret* Committee for overseeing the development of psychoanalysis" provide an answer (quoted from a letter from Freud to Ferenczi dated 12 August 1912; CF, 404). In July 1912 Jones proposed to Ferenczi that an "Old Guard" or secret society be set up to protect against potential dissension which might betray Freud's basic tenets. Quite enthusiastic about the idea of such a secret association, Freud wrote to Jones on 1 August 1912:

> What took hold of my imagination immediately is your idea of a secret council composed of the best and most trustworthy among our men to take care of the further development of psycho-analysis and defend the cause against personalities and accidents when I am no more . . . I know there is a boyish and perhaps romantic element too in this conception, but perhaps it could be adapted to meet the necessities of reality. I will give my fancy free play and leave to you the part of censor.
>
> I daresay it would make living and dying easier for me if I knew of such an association existing to watch over my creation.
>
> First of all: This committee would have to be *strictly secret* in its existence and its action. It could be composed of you, Ferenczi and [Otto] Rank among whom the idea was generated. [Hans] Sachs, in whom my confidence is unlimited in spite of the shortness of our acquaintance—and [Karl] Abraham could be called next, but only under the condition of all of you consenting. I had better be left outside of your conditions and pledges: to be sure I will keep the utmost secrecy and be thankful for all you communicate to me.
>
> (LW, 153–154; the emphasis is Freud's)

The part of censor Freud bestowed thus on Jones in 1912 is contrary to the concept of censorship in psychoanalytic theory. Construed as the mental agency responsible for the distortion of dream thoughts, censorship is destined to yield to interpretation.

Freud sees the silence underlying dreams as one ultimately seeking revelation. How can we explain the discrepancy between censorship as a psychoanalytic concept and censorship as a historical feature of the psychoanalytic movement? The disparity between the two types of censorship—the one urging disclosure, the other concealment—could not be greater. The censor must never betray the trust placed in him as a warden of silence. In contrast to the analyst, who attempts with the patient to overcome repression, the censor resists the restoration of any deleted material because it would reveal a secret pact.

Given his disputes with Jung just then, Freud's apprehension for the safety of his system might seem somewhat reasonable in 1912–1913. But historical documents were being suppressed in the 1950s, at a time when the Freudian establishment was enjoying its golden age and all threats, at least in the West, to eradicate the psychoanalytic movement had vanished. Therefore any censorship of documents at that time and since is certainly not due to external dangers and has to be regarded as part of the internal historical topography of psychoanalysis itself. Here is the paradox. The purpose of Freudian psychoanalysis is to detect and dispel all forms of mental censorship, in individuals and society at large. But the censorship of the founding documents of Freudianism seeks to impose a barrier not to be removed.

The Setbacks of Catharsis:
Emmy von N.

The paradox of censorship in Freudian theory and in the history of the psychoanalytic movement will emerge more clearly if we turn to an early clinical work of Freud's in which he assumes the unusual role of the "censor" who deletes traumas. The case of Emmy von N., the first Freud records in *Studies on Hysteria,* foreshadows the tension between lifting and imposing censorship.

In 1889 Emmy von N. was to represent Freud's first attempt at applying the hypnotic-cathartic method of treatment he had learned from his older colleague Dr. Josef Breuer, a method that allowed patients to release their pent-up psychic tension under hypnosis. "On May 1, 1889 I took on the case of a lady of about forty years of age . . . She was a hysteric and could be put into a state of somnambulism with the greatest ease . . . I decided that I would make use of Breuer's technique of investigation under hypnosis . . . This was my first attempt at handling that therapeutic method" (S, 48). Actually, Freud combined several therapeutic

techniques, as he was under the simultaneous influence of two
other contemporary approaches, Hyppolyte Bernheim's method
of didactic suggestion and Pierre Janet's procedure of weakening
painful emotions. However, the technique of memory extinction,
a specifically Freudian "therapeutic method," had little to do with
any other contemporary form of psychotherapy and least of all
with Breuer's cathartic method. Contrary to the stated objectives
of Breuerian catharsis and subsequently of Freudian psychoanalysis (the working out of traumas and/or conflicts in the transfer-
ential relationship between patient and analyst), we see in the case
history of Emmy von N. the permanent deletion of the patient's
traumatic memories. Whereas both catharsis and psychoanalysis
aim to provide therapeutic tools for coming into contact with
oneself, Freud used a technique of disconnection, removing his
patient's ability to know her own past.

> I requested her, under hypnosis, to talk, which, after some
> effort, she succeeded in doing . . . This series of traumatic
> precipitating causes which she produced in answer to my
> question . . . was clearly ready to hand in her memory . . .
> At the end of each separate story she twitched all over and
> took on a look of fear and horror. At the end of the last one
> she opened her mouth wide and panted for breath. The
> words in which she described the terrifying subject-matter
> of her experience were pronounced with difficulty and be-
> tween gaps. Afterwards her features became peaceful.
>
> (S, 52)

In reply to a question she told me that while she was
describing these scenes she saw them before her, in a plastic
form and in their natural colours. She said that in general
she thought of these experiences very often and had done
so in the last few days. Whenever this happened she saw
these scenes with all the vividness of reality . . . My therapy

consists in wiping away these pictures, so that she is no longer able to see them before her. To give support to my suggestion I stroked her several times over the eyes.

(S, 53)

I had asked her the origin of her stammering . . . I further learnt from her that the stammer had begun immediately after the first of these two occasions . . . I extinguished her plastic memory of these scenes . . . Finding her disposed to be communicative, I asked her what further events in her life had frightened her so much that they left her with plastic memories. She replied by giving me a collection of such experiences: . . . How she had nursed her sick brother and he had such fearful attacks as a result of the morphine and had terrified her and seized hold of her. I remembered that she had already mentioned this experience this morning, and, as an experiment, I asked her on what other occasions this "seizing hold" had happened. To my agreeable surprise she made a long pause this time before answering and then asked doubtfully "My little girl?" She was quite unable to recall the other two occasions (see above). My prohibition— my expunging of her memories—had therefore been effective. (S, 57–59)

I saw that I had come to the root of her constant fear of surprises and I asked further instances of this. She went on: how they had a friend staying at her home . . . how she had been so ill after her mother's death . . . and lastly, how, on the journey . . . I wiped out all these memories, woke her up and assured her she would sleep well tonight. (S, 59)

Under hypnosis I asked her what event in her life had produced the most lasting effect on her and came up most often in her memory. Her husband's death, she said. I got her to describe this event in full detail, and this she did with every sign of the deepest emotion . . . I made it impossible for her to see any of these melancholy things again, not only by wiping out her memories of them in their *plastic* form but by removing her whole recollection of them, as though they had never been present in her mind.   (S, 60–61)

[Emmy] von N.'s psychical situation can be characterized . . . Her memory exhibited a lively activity which, sometimes spontaneously, sometimes in response to a contemporary stimulus . . . , brought her traumas with the accompanying affects bit by bit into her present-day consciousness. My therapeutic procedure was based on the course of this activity of her memory and endeavored day by day to resolve and get rid of whatever that particular day had brought to the surface, till the accessible stock of her pathological memories seemed to be exhausted.   (S, 90)

Breuer's cathartic method provided patients with diverse means—speech, convulsion, tears, rage—of coming into contact with themselves and their traumatic recollections. Freud's therapy of Emmy von N. consisted of deletion. The result was the exact opposite of Breuer's: it severed all contact with the forgotten and even the consciously remembered past. Freud knew that the richest store of Emmy von N.'s traumatic memories could come to light only in the somnambulistic state. Since he eradicated her recollections under hypnosis, they never managed to reach her waking consciousness.

Freud indicated that he had hoped to master Breuer's cathartic method through his analysis of Emmy von N. and even noted some dissatisfaction with not having been able to pursue Breuer's method systematically enough (S, 48). Yet his recurring metaphors of deletion would seem to contradict his stated intentions. "I wiped out all these memories"; "I made it impossible for her to see these melancholy things again . . . by removing her whole recollection of them"; "my prohibition—my expunging of her memories"; "I extinguished her plastic memory"; "I took this memory-picture away"; "in a few weeks we were able to dispose of these memories too," and so on. These metaphors describe a mechanism of extinction, not a procedure for enhancing contact with oneself. The effect of Freud's very uncathartic method was that Emmy von N. forgot the most important events of her life.

"When, as much as eighteen months later, I saw Frau Emmy again in a relatively good state of health, she complained that there were a number of most important moments in her life of which she had only the vaguest memory. She regarded this as evidence of a weakening of her memory, and I had to be careful not to tell her the cause of this particular instance of amnesia" (S, 61). Had Freud been working with the complete idea of catharsis, his treatment of Emmy von N. would have (1) led to the purgative release of her pent-up emotions; (2) ended the amnesia that had cut off the painful and pathogenic ideas from associative communication with the rest of the patient's mental life; (3) thereby bringing the traumatic memories to consciousness; (4) with the ultimate aim of permanently dissipating the symptoms that derive from emotions connected with forgotten traumatic events. The successive stages of recall under hypnosis, release of tension, the restoration of the free-flowing continuity of mental life, and finally the disappearance of the symptom characterize Breuer's cathartic method, set forth repeatedly in *Studies on Hysteria,* for example at the end of the "Preliminary Communication" (co-written by Freud): "It will now be understood how it is that the psycho-therapeutic procedure which we have described in these pages has a curative effect. *It brings an end to the operative force of the idea which was not abreacted in the first instance, by allowing its strangulated affect to find a way through speech; and it subjects it to associative correction by introducing it into normal consciousness*" (S, 17; emphasis in original).

Freud stressed this last point again at the end of case number 3: "The therapeutic process in this case consisted in compelling the psychic group that had been split off to unite once more with the ego-consciousness" (S, 124). Moreover, in an 1888 encyclopedic article entitled "Hysteria" (a year before his treatment of Emmy von N.) Freud had singled out this very aspect to illustrate the chief characteristic of Breuer's method of treatment: "[Hypnosis] is even more effective if we adopt a method first practised by Joseph Breuer in Vienna and lead the patient under hypnosis to the psychical prehistory of the ailment and compel him to acknowledge the psychical occasion on which the disorder in question originated" ("Hysteria," SE 1:56).

Freud's procedure of deletion led to a unique relationship between patient and therapist. Entirely without the patient's knowledge—and therefore in quite a different way from a pact of professional secrecy—Freud became the sole repository for Emmy von N.'s expunged memories. As for Emmy herself, she was far from suspecting that Freud had kept her memories for himself. All she does is offer the incident of her forgetting two words describing secret meeting places in ancient Rome:

> She told me of a visit she had paid to the Roman catacombs, but could not recall two technical terms; nor could I help her with them. Immediately afterwards I asked her under hypnosis which words she had in mind. But she did not know them in hypnosis either. So I said to her: "Don't bother about them any more now, but when you are in the garden to-morrow between five and six in the afternoon—nearer six than five—they will suddenly occur to you." Next evening, while we were talking about something which had no connection with catacombs, she suddenly burst out: "Crypt, doctor, and columbarium." "Ah, those are the words you couldn't think of yesterday. When did they occur to you?" "In the garden this afternoon." (S, 98).

In this conversation, the words crypt and columbarium refer to Rome in Emmy von N.'s eyes. But was she not also describing

Freud, her master of memories, as "doctor crypt and columbarium," the place where the secret burial of her past had occurred?[1]

To conclude that Freud became Emmy von N.'s crypt is either a metaphorical abuse of language or a mystery. And if mystery there is, it will seem all the more significant once we notice an analogy between Freud, the secret warden of his patient's memories in 1889, and Jones, the secret guardian of censored documents in 1957, documents whose very existence he had denied.

The secret committee, established for the "supervision of the development of psychoanalysis," is a direct corollary in 1912 to the secret depository Freud had created more than twenty years earlier during his psychotherapy of Emmy von N. In her case Freud had performed the twofold action of wiping out her memories and of depositing them in a secret storehouse—in himself. The committee too represents the creation of a secret enclave within the larger boundaries of a publicly proclaimed International Psychoanalytic Association (founded in 1910). Obliged by its members to remain "strictly secret in its existence," the committee was called upon to function as the highest authority legitimizing the definition of psychoanalysis. Yet, by virtue of this pledge of secrecy, psychoanalysis withdrew in 1912 from the very domain it had sought to open. Rather curiously, but certainly not without reason, the seven rings owned by the committee's members allegorize the same structure: "On May 25, 1913 Freud celebrated the event [the creation of the committee] by presenting us each with an antique Greek intaglio from his collection which we then got mounted in a gold ring. Freud himself had long carried such a ring, a Greek-Roman intaglio with the head of Jupiter, and when some seven years later [Max] Eitingon was also given one there were the 'Seven Rings'" (LW, 2:154). Each intaglio Freud presented to his paladins became recessed in a ring just as the secret committee was set within the International Psychoanalytic Association.

Neutralizing Constructive Criticism: Freud Faced with Ferenczi's Research on Trauma

Twenty years after the creation of the secret committee in 1912, an unexpected development underscored the continuing importance of censorship in the history of psychoanalysis. It was Freud's uncompromising refusal to acknowledge the value of the inquiries of Sándor Ferenczi, his intimate friend and fervent disciple, into trauma. Ferenczi's interest from 1929 on in the traumatic events of early childhood set off a bitterly personal reaction in Freud. In his letters to Ferenczi, Freud did not engage in a substantive exchange of views but gave vent to his ill humor instead, expressing his all-encompassing disapproval, his near despair, at seeing his friend slip from his control. Ferenczi's conceptual departures occurred almost in spite of himself, though, under the compelling influence of his clinical insights. Freud's disappointment culminated in his attempt to prevent or postpone the publication of Ferenczi's final paper, "Confusion of Tongues between Adults and the Child" (1932).

For the last decade or so, scholars have begun studying Freud's rejection of the late Ferenczi. Ever since 1953 we have had a glimpse into some of the circumstances, albeit in a fragmentary, tendentious, and even spiteful representation, given by Jones in his biography of Freud. The Freud-Ferenczi letters have since completed the picture for us along with the investigations of Jeffrey Masson in *The Assault on Truth*, Barbro Sylwan, and Maria Torok (in the French journal *Cahiers Confrontation* 12, 1984). We consider Freud's rejection of Ferenczi a crucial instance of censorship in the historical topography of psychoanalysis. (In the following discussion we will quote from the not-yet-published portion of the Freud-Ferenczi correspondence. We thank Judith Dupont for giving us access from 1981 on to the complete unpublished letters.)

As Freud put it in a letter to Ferenczi (dated 11 January 1933), the friendship between the two men extended far beyond mutual understanding to "an intimate community of life, feeling, and interests." It is also widely recognized that Ferenczi became the most enthusiastic and most admired proponent of Freudianism in his lifetime, distinguishing himself by his untiring efforts to disseminate and broaden his teacher's discoveries. Founder of the International Psychoanalytic Association in 1910, Ferenczi also proposed the introduction of the so-called training analysis as a necessary stage in the education of future analysts. Countless ties of friendship, thought, and professional endeavor thus united Freud and Ferenczi, yet a far-reaching disagreement concerning the etiological significance of trauma drove an increasingly bitter wedge between them from 1929 until Ferenczi's death in 1933.

Because of his implicit loyalty to Freud, Ferenczi was quite slow to realize that he was recasting some of Freud's theories and especially his therapeutic approach. Despite his own distress, oc- casionally mentioned to Freud himself in their correspondence, Ferenczi did come to disagree with several of his teacher's basic tenets. He charged, for example, that psychoanalysis had moved away from its initial inquiries into individual trauma and privileged more and more the role of fantasy, the universal Oedipus and castration complexes, and the conflicts arising among the psychic agencies (ego, id, and superego). Actually, Ferenczi never wanted to part with any of Freud's mature theories from the 1920s and early 1930s; he merely sought to complete them with a parallel theory, taking into account real events and their potentially traumatic psychological effects. He attempted to revive and strengthen an already existing though long-neglected tradition of psychoanalytic research into trauma, a tradition he saw embodied in Breuer's and Freud's *Studies on Hysteria* (1895). However, Freud's reaction to Ferenczi's interest in trauma proved nothing short of explosively emotional. He wielded his authority as the founder of psychoanalysis and his influence as Ferenczi's sometime analyst to scold him, going so far as to volunteer tendentious psychological interpretations of Ferenczi's behavior.

In his letters to Freud and Max Eitingon, Ferenczi urged from 1929 on the necessity of expanding the contemporary psychoanalytic framework to include the less-understood reality of those psychotic patients who suffered severe psychological shocks. Excerpts follow (unless otherwise stated, translations from the German are ours):

Ferenczi's letter to Freud dated 29 December 1929:

My true gift is after all in research; devoid of all personal ambition, I am given to studying my cases with double curiosity, so to speak, without conceiving any rigid opinions; experiences have accumulated, taking me in a certain direction, to which I alluded in my paper at Oxford ["Principle of Relaxation and Neo-Catharsis," 1929].

This is what I can tell you in a brief summary:

1. In all cases where I went far enough, I found the traumatic-hysterical grounds of illness.

2. When the patients and I reached that point, the therapeutic impact proved much greater . . .

3. I have slowly come around to the critical point of view that psychoanalysis has restricted itself to the analysis of either obsessional neuroses or the neurosis of character, while it has neglected the organic-hysterical foundations of psychoanalysis itself. The reason for this is the overvaluation of fantasy and the underestimation of traumatic reality in pathogenesis.

I do not know whether you can consider this as an "oppositional tendency." I believe that this would be unjustified. It is simply a tendency based on experience.

Ferenczi's letter to Freud dated 17 January 1930:

An exaggerated concern for your health has prevented me for a long time from telling you about my reservations concerning the narrow-minded development of psychoanalysis . . . I do not agree with you, for example, that the therapeutic process should be neglected or considered less important, or that, simply because it seems uninteresting to us, we have the right to neglect it.

Ferenczi's letter to Freud dated 15 February 1930:

I would like to keep my impressions about *Civilization and Discontents* for a visit in Vienna . . . I would only suggest something in one place (no doubt from the traumatic point of view). Would it not be wiser to hold fast to the individual, traumatic nature or origin of moral conscience and of neurosis . . . ?

Ferenczi's letter to Freud dated 20 July 1930:

This subjective factor has made me receptive, I think, to psychological processes among our neurotics, processes that occur in moments of real or supposed mortal danger. This is indeed the path that led me to reinstate the apparently outdated (and, in any case long-neglected) trauma theory.

Ferenczi's letter to Freud dated 31 May 1931 (this letter includes the abstract of a proposed lecture by Ferenczi, an abstract originally sent to Max Eitingon):

Dr. Ferenczi's paper:

1. *Do dreams have a second function?*

If we base ourselves on the experiences of those psycho-analytic sessions in which a deep relaxation [of the patient] occurs—this [relaxation] promotes the repetition of trau-matic scenes—as well as on the analysis of dreams, we might conjecture that [apart from wish-fulfillment] both sleep and dreams also attempt to unburden the psychic apparatus by reexperiencing daily residues or the residues of life.

2. *A possible extension of our metapsychological views:*

Freud's metapsychological constructions result from expe-riences with neurotics (repression). It is equally legitimate to take seriously, as a form of psychoanalytic reality, the rather different and yet nearly universal mechanisms that lurk behind the [mental] productions of psychotics and traumatized people (fragmentation and atomization of the personality; sequestering).

In three articles written between 1929 and 1932 ("The Prin-ciples of Relaxation and Neocatharsis," "Child-Analysis in the Analysis of Adults," "Confusion of Tongues between Adults and the Child"), Ferenczi devised highly personal techniques of sym-pathetic receptiveness in order to foster the reemergence of his patients' past trauma; he also gave a detailed analysis of the psychological mechanisms attendant upon traumatic shock. Freud's reaction to Ferenczi's theoretical and clinical correctives was invariably negative and final. Whether Ferenczi imparted his ideas in the somewhat faltering style of gestating thoughts in private letters or in the more definitive form of conference papers, Freud rejected Ferenczi without refuting his claims. Freud attempted to dissuade him, to convince him with emotional arguments of the baselessness of his ideas.

Freud's letter to Ferenczi dated 18 September 1931:

> There can be no doubt that . . . you keep away from me more and more. I am not saying and I hope that you're not turning away from me. I ascribe it to fate like so many other things and I know that it is not my fault, and even lately I have preferred no one to you. I note with regret—and it is an expression of your inner dissatisfaction—that you are trying to go in all kinds of directions that will lead to no desirable goal for me.
>
> Yet I have always respected your autonomy, as you yourself acknowledge; I am ready to wait patiently until you decide to change by yourself. Yours could be a case of third puberty, after which you will no doubt reach maturity.

Rather often Freud suggested in this way to Ferenczi that his clinical and theoretical interest in trauma derived in the final analysis from personal and unresolved neurotic factors. He expected Ferenczi to be reasonable again, to stop acting like a recalcitrant child, rebelling against others, especially Freud.

Freud's categorical rejection of and personal bitterness over Ferenczi's scientific inquiries culminated with Ferenczi's participation in the International Psychoanalytic Association's annual convention in 1932. Ferenczi's paper to be delivered there, "The Confusion of Tongues between Adults and the Child," speaks of the potentially traumatic clash between the child's emotions (dominated by tenderness) and those of the adult (dominated instead by passion), the latter conveying brutality to the child.

The collision of the two emotional worlds takes on catastrophic proportions, according to Ferenczi, when, submitting to the adult's passionate advances, sexually and emotionally immature children identify with their aggressor and become the unconscious playthings of their aggressor's will. Ferenczi studies, in this identification, the pathological consequences for children, for example their radical and disturbing loss of the memory of the trauma. In a letter to Ferenczi dated 20 October 1932, Freud recalled the apprehension he had felt on meeting Ferenczi a few weeks before the congress; he feared that Ferenczi's speech would create a scandal and begged him to postpone its publication. It becomes clear from an earlier letter by Ferenczi that Freud had considered the paper harmful both for psychoanalysis and for Ferenczi himself.

Freud's letter to Ferenczi dated 2 October 1932 (published in part by Masson in *The Assault on Truth*):

> My request to put off the publication by one year was primarily in your interest. I did not want to give up the hope that in your further work you would come to recognize the technical shortcomings of your procedure and the limited truthfulness of your results. You seemed to concede as much, but I relieve you, of course, of your promise and abdicate all influence, which I do not actually command anyway. I no longer think that you will correct your mistake as I did mine a generation ago.

In this letter Freud views Ferenczi's traumatological studies from the 1930s as if they concerned himself before the turn of the previous century. In September 1897 Freud attempted to change thoroughly his earlier convictions about the etiology of hysteria. His new position was to be that what patients pass off as their childhood realities are in fact their fantasies. Thus, in Freud's eyes, Ferenczi quite simply regressed to an outdated stage of Freud's own career, a stage marked by etiological errors duly corrected since then. So Ferenczi overestimates reality and underestimates fantasy, as Freud had done some thirty-five years earlier. In other words, Ferenczi in his middle years appears to have been lured into the younger Freud's own mistake, with the difference that he refuses to apply Freud's correction.

Freud's letter to Eitingon dated 28 August 1933 (quoted from AT, 182):

> His source is what patients tell him when he manages to put them into what he himself calls a state similar to hypnosis. He then takes what he hears as revelations, but what one really gets are the fantasies of patients about their childhood, and not the [real] story. My first great etiological error also arose in this very way.[2]

In his historical works—especially *On the History of the Psycho-Analytical Movement* (1914) and *An Autobiographical Study* (1925)—Freud did in fact give the impression that he had rejected in one fell sweep and forever his erstwhile theories. However, as we have seen, several of his theoretical and clinical works, as well as his correspondence with Fliess (see Chapter 2) show Freud oscillating; they tell that Freud's abandonment of his seduction theory and its subsequent replacement by the idea of infantile sexual fantasies fluctuated for decades as he periodically returned to his former position. From the letters Freud wrote to Ferenczi, Jones, and Eitingon between 1931 and 1933, we might indeed think that Freud has finally overcome his bafflement over the respective status of reality and fantasy. But his highly charged attitude toward Ferenczi proves the contrary. Freud blamed Ferenczi for overvaluing reality at the expense of fantasy. Ferenczi reversed the roles: it is Freud who overvalues fantasy at the expense of traumatic reality.

While the theoretical disagreement appears crystal clear to the impartial observer, Freud's refusal to enter into any substantive discussion seems much less so. We think that Freud's extraordinary unwillingness to admit the potential fruitfulness of a theoretical position different from his current one is understandable only in the retrospective light of his own obstinate etiological hesitation—no doubt violently shaken up by Ferenczi's decisive traumatological research. No wonder, since Ferenczi was his most trusted theoretical companion and his most beloved personal friend.[3]

The censorship of Ferenczi will take on a rather complex hue if we consider it in the light of Freud's own early investigations of psychic trauma. The synoptic confrontation of key passages from Ferenczi's "Confusion of Tongues between Adults and the Child" (1932) and Freud's "Aetiology of Hysteria" (1896) will demonstrate a striking convergence of the two men's views. (Our quotes will also include two other texts by Ferenczi as well as a letter to Freud. Occasionally we will modernize the translation of Ferenczi's texts, published in 1955.) Following this unusual dialogue, we will ask: Did Ferenczi become, in Freud's heart, a detestable reminder of his own vacillation between real and fantasized trauma?

Traumatic Events in Childhood

FREUD

Sexual experiences in childhood consisting in stimulation of the genitals, coitus-like acts, and so on, must therefore be recognized, in the last analysis, as being the traumas which lead to a hysterical reaction. (A, 206–207)

In all eighteen cases . . . I have . . . come to learn of sexual experiences of this kind in childhood . . . it is a question of assaults . . . instances of abuse, mostly practised on female children by adults who were strangers . . . The second group consists of the much more numerous cases where some adult looking after the child—a nursery maid or governess or tutor, or, unhappily all too often, a close relative—has initiated the child into sexual intercourse and has maintained a regular love relationship with it . . . which has often lasted for years.   (A, 207–208)

I therefore put forward the thesis that at the bottom of every case of hysteria there are *one or more occurrences of premature sexual experience,* occurrences which belong to the earliest years of childhood but which can be reproduced through the work of psycho-analysis in spite of the intervening decades. I believe that this is an important finding, the discovery of a *caput Nili* [source of the Nile] in neuropathology.

(A, 203)

And since infantile experiences with a sexual content could after all only exert a psychical effect through their *memory-traces,* would not this view be a welcome amplification of the finding of psycho-analysis which tells us that *hysterical symptoms can only arise with the co-operation of memories?*

(A, 202)

FERENCZI

I obtained above all new corroborative evidence for my supposition that the trauma, as the pathogenic factor cannot be valued highly enough. Even children of very respectable, sincerely puritanical families fall victim to real violence or rape . . . Either it is the parents who try to find a substitute gratification in this pathological way for their frustration, or it is people thought to be trustworthy such as relatives (uncles, aunts, grandparents), governesses or servants, who misuse the ignorance and the innocence of the child.

(FC, 161)

The real rape of girls who have hardly grown out of the age of infants, similar sexual acts of mature women with boys, and also enforced homosexual acts, are more frequent occurrences than has hitherto been assumed.

(FC, 161–162)

The recollections which neocatharsis evoked or corroborated lent great significance to the original traumatic factor . . . Accordingly, no analysis can be regarded . . . as complete unless we have succeeded in penetrating to the traumatic material . . . Having given due consideration to fantasy as a pathogenic factor, I have, of late been forced more and more to deal with the pathogenic trauma itself.

(FC, 120)

In all cases where I went far enough, I found the traumatic-hysterical grounds of illness.

(Letter to Freud, 25 December 1929)

Heredity or Trauma?

FREUD

Where there had been a relation between two children I was sometimes able to prove that the boy—who, here too, played the part of the aggressor—had previously been seduced . . . The foundation for a neurosis would accordingly always be laid in childhood by adults, and the children themselves would transfer to one another the disposition to fall ill from hysteria later . . . Supposing, then, ten or fifteen years later several members of the younger generation of the family are found to be ill, might not this appearance of a family neurosis naturally lead to the false supposition that a hereditary disposition is present where there is only a *pseudo-heredity*? (A, 208–209)

FERENCZI

By that I mean the recent, more emphatic stress on the traumatic factors in the pathogenesis of the neuroses which had been unjustly neglected in recent years. Insufficient exploration of the external factor leads to the danger of resorting prematurely to explanations . . . in terms of "disposition" and "constitution."   (FC, 156)

It became evident that this [trauma] is far more rarely the result of a constitutional hypersensitivity in children . . . than of really improper . . . or actually cruel treatment.

(FC, 120–121)

Therapy

FREUD

The reaction of hysterics is only apparently exaggerated; it is bound to appear exaggerated to us only because we only know a small part of the motives from which it arises.   (A, 217)

It is not the latest slight—which, in itself, is minimal—that produces the fit of crying, the outburst of despair or the attempt at suicide, . . . [but] the small slight of the present moment has aroused . . . the memory of a serious slight in childhood which has never been overcome . . . Finally, the problem of the hysterogenic points is of the same kind. If you touch a particular spot . . . you awaken a memory which may start off a convulsive attack.   (A, 217–218)

If we try . . . to induce the symptoms of a hysteria to make themselves heard as witnesses to the history of the origin of the illness, we must take our start from Josef Breuer's momentous discovery: *the symptoms of hysteria . . . are determined by certain experiences of the patient's which have oper-*

ated in a traumatic fashion and which are being reproduced in his psychical life in the form of mnemic symbols . . . Having thus located the scene, we remove the symptom by bringing about, during the reproduction of the traumatic scene, a subsequent correction of the psychical course of events which took place at the time. (A, 192–193)

FERENCZI

After we had succeeded in a somewhat deeper manner than before in creating an atmosphere of confidence between physician and patient and in securing a fuller freedom of affect, hysterical physical symptoms would suddenly make their appearance, often for the first time in an analysis extending over years. These symptoms included paresthesias and spasms, definitely localized, violent emotional movements, like miniature hysterical attacks, sudden alterations of the state of consciousness, slight vertigo and a clouding of consciousness often with subsequent amnesia of what had taken place . . . In certain cases these hysterical attacks actually assumed the character of *trances,* in which fragments of the past were relived . . . I was able to question them and received important information about dissociated parts of the personality. Without any such intention on my part . . . unusual states of consciousness manifested themselves . . . Willy-nilly, one was forced to compare them with the phenomena of the Breuer-Freud *catharsis.* (FC, 118–119)

Pathogenesis or the Origins of Psychic Trauma

FREUD

The outbreak of hysteria may almost invariably be traced to a *psychical conflict* arising through an incompatible idea setting in action a *defence* on the part of the ego and calling up a demand for repression . . . *The defence achieves its purpose of thrusting the incompatible idea out of consciousness if there are infantile sexual scenes present in the (hitherto normal) subject in the form of unconscious memories.*

(A, 210–211)

With our patients, those memories are never conscious; but we cure them of their hysteria by transforming their unconscious memories of the infantile scenes into conscious ones.

(A, 211)

All the singular conditions under which the ill-matched pair conduct their love-relations—on the one hand the adult, . . . who is . . . armed with complete authority and the right to punish, and can exchange the one role for the other to the uninhibited satisfaction of his moods, and on the other hand the child, who in his helplessness is at the mercy of this arbitrary will, who is prematurely aroused to every kind of sensibility and exposed to every sort of disappointment, and whose performance of the sexual activities assigned to him is often interrupted by his imperfect control of his natural needs—all these grotesque and yet tragic incongruities reveal themselves as stamped upon the later development of the individual and of his neurosis, in countless permanent effects which deserve to be traced in the greatest detail.

(A, 215)

What, then, determines whether the infantile sexual scenes which have remained unconscious will later on, when the other pathogenic factors are super-added, give rise to hysterical or to obsessional neurosis or even to paranoia?

(A, 219)

So far, I have observed that obsessions can be regularly shown to be disguised and transformed *self-reproaches about acts of sexual aggression in childhood* . . . From this I might conclude that the character of the infantile scenes—whether they were experienced with pleasure or only passively—has a determining influence on the later neurosis.   (A, 220)

FERENCZI

It is difficult to imagine the behaviour and the emotions of children after such violence. One would expect the first impulse to be . . . hatred, disgust, and energetic refusal. "No, no, I do not want it, . . . it hurts, leave me alone," this or something similar would be the immediate reaction if it had not been paralyzed by enormous anxiety. These children feel physically and morally helpless, their personalities are not sufficiently consolidated in order to be able to protest, even if only in thought, for the overpowering force and authority of the adult makes them dumb and can rob them of their senses. *The same anxiety, however, if it reaches . . . a maximum, compels them to subordinate themselves like automata to the will of the aggressor, to divine and gratify each one of his desires; completely oblivious of themselves, they identify with the aggressor* . . . The most important change, produced in the child's mind by anxiety and the fear-ridden identification with the adult partner, is *the introjection of the guilt feelings of the adult;* this makes the hitherto harmless play appear as a punishable offence.

(FC, 162; translation slightly modified)

This process allows us to observe the mechanism of a trauma's genesis. First, there is complete paralysis of all spontaneity, including any and all activity of thinking and, on the physical side, even a condition resembling shock or coma may result . . . we shall find that children, when they feel abandoned, lose all interest in life or, as we might say with Freud, they turn their aggressive impulses against themselves. Sometimes this process goes so far that patients begin to have sensations of sinking and dying. They will turn deadly pale, or fall into a state like fainting . . . What we here see taking place is the reproduction of the mental and physical agony that follows upon incomprehensible and intolerable suffering.   (FC, 137–138; translation slightly modified)

If children recover from such an attack, they feel enormously confused, actually their personality is already split—they are innocent and guilty at the same time—and their confidence in the testimony of their own senses is broken. Moreover, the harsh behaviour of the adult partner, tormented and made angry by his remorse, makes children all the more conscious of their guilt and shame. The perpetrator almost always behaves as though nothing had happened and consoles himself with the thought: "Oh, it is only a child, it knows nothing, and will forget it all." Quite frequently after such events, the seducer adheres to a strict sense of morality or becomes religious, endeavoring to save the child's soul by severity. Usually the confidential relation to a second adult—[for example] . . . the mother—is not intimate enough for the child to find help there; timid attempts to this end are repulsed by her . . . The misused child changes into a mechanical, obedient automaton, or becomes defiant, but is unable to account for the reasons of his defiance. His sexual life remains undeveloped or assumes perverted forms.

(FC, 162–163; translation modified)

The Genuineness of Childhood Trauma

FREUD

Doubts about the genuineness of the infantile scenes can, however, be deprived of their force here and now by more than one argument. In the first place, the behaviour of patients while they are reproducing these infantile experiences is in every respect incompatible with the assumption that the scenes are anything else than a reality which is being felt with distress and reproduced with the greatest reluctance. Before they come for analysis the patients know nothing about these scenes . . . While they are recalling these infantile experiences to consciousness, they suffer under the most violent sensations, of which they are ashamed and which they try to conceal; and, even after they have gone through them once more in such a convincing manner, they still attempt to withhold belief from them . . . Why should patients assure me so emphatically of their unbelief, if what they want to discredit is something which—from whatever motive—they themselves have invented? (A, 204)

In the second place, patients sometimes describe as harmless events whose significance they obviously do not understand, since they would be bound otherwise to be horrified by them. Or again, they mention details, without laying any stress on them, which only someone of experience in life can understand and appreciate as subtle traits of reality.

(A, 205)

FERENCZI

The immediate objection—that these are only sexual fantasies of the child, a kind of hysterical lying—is unfortunately made invalid by the number of confessions about assaults upon children that had been committed by patients now in analysis. (FC, 161; translation slightly modified)

Hysterical fantasies do not lie when they tell us that parents and other adults do indeed go to great lengths in their passionately erotic relation with children.

(FC, 121; translation slightly modified)

The highly important assumption . . . is that *the weak and undeveloped personality* [of the child] *reacts to sudden unpleasure not by defence, but by an anxiety-ridden identification . . . with the menacing person or aggressor.* Only with the help of this hypothesis can I understand why my patients refuse so obstinately to follow my advice and react to unjust or unkind treatment with . . . hatred and defence. One part of their personality, possibly its very nucleus, got stuck at a certain level . . . Thus arises a kind of personality . . . that lacks the ability to assert itself in the face of displeasure.

(FC, 163; translation modified)

The patient then tells us of the inappropriate actions and reactions of adults to traumatic shocks suffered in childhood. Probably the worst way of dealing with such situations is to deny their existence, to assert that nothing happened, that nothing actually hurt the child, or for children to be actually scolded or beaten when they manifest a traumatic paralysis of thought or movement. These are the kinds of treatment that make the trauma pathogenic.

(FC, 138; translation modified)

Was it because of his demonstration of the undiminished validity and continuing relevance of Freud's forsaken views on the reality of infantile seductions that Ferenczi became unbearable to Freud after 1929? The conceptual affinity, the emotional closeness between Freud (in 1896) and Ferenczi (in 1932) lead us to think so. At a time when Freud, gravely affected by his cancer of the jaw, was thinking only of his legacy, the all too convincing restoration of his outdated trauma theory must have threatened to rekindle his etiological afflictions of yesteryear. Rather than yield again to his own vacillation, did Freud prefer to quash it once and for all—*in Ferenczi*? Wanting to weaken the late Ferenczi's research, did Freud actually censor himself? The result was an uncommon interpersonal situation. From 1932 on, Freud carried on a portion of his characteristic vacillation under the guise of Ferenczi. As a result, Freud was finally free to consolidate for posterity an unshakable body of doctrine. This became suddenly possible because Ferenczi, the beloved grand vizier, had adopted as his own Freud's deserted seduction theory.

A brief historical sketch is necessary here. Some pioneers of psychoanalysis, such as Ferenczi, have been all but banned. The institutional ostracism of Ferenczi after his death (despite Freud's eloquent homage in his eulogy of his departed friend in 1933) has driven his works to a nearly underground existence, marked by long and insidious exclusions or silences. Ferenczi's complete works, first published in English in 1955 thanks to Michael Balint, his Hungarian disciple, became available in French only in 1982 (after two and a half decades of efforts by Judith Dupont and, initially, by Nicolas Abraham).

In addition, one could show that significant portions of subsequent psychoanalytic research (for example in D. W. Winnicott's work) rely on Ferenczi's key ideas, without his being acknowledged as the primary source. This is so for two reasons. Second- and third-generation psychoanalysts either tacitly followed the institutional exclusion of Ferenczi's work or quite simply did not know it because of that exclusion. Hence it is quite possible for a British analyst to introduce as his own, in the 1990s, ideas and clinical attitudes reflected on and described by Ferenczi in the 1920s. It is also important to note here that within the ranks of the International Psychoanalytic Association itself there exists at the present time something resembling a sustained interest in Ferenczi's works. This recent desire to revive Ferenczi after sixty years of silence is somewhat strategic. At a juncture when the scientific credibility and therapeutic usefulness of psychoanalysis are being assailed on all sides, the discovery of a "new" pioneer might return the psychoanalytic institution to rosier days. Yet, in a sense, the motivation for this belated recognition of one of the most fruitfully critical views of classical Freudianism does not matter. The fact remains that the nascent discussion of Ferenczi's work can help transform the whole of psychoanalysis.

The attempt to suppress Ferenczi's original research, the censorship of the Freud-Fliess letters, the creation of a secret committee, and Emmy von N.'s clinical case of deletion mark a hitherto unnoticed thread of continuity in the development of psychoanalysis. However, these transverse developments fall outside the domain of psychoanalytic theory as it was known in 1957, the year of Ludwig Marcuse's ill-fated request to gain access to Freud's expurgated correspondence. Neither the *secret* existence of the committee nor *the expunging of* Emmy von N.'s memories can be understood in terms of the Freudian concept of dynamic repression. These phenomena also do not fit the Freudian model of a mental topography whose repressions and internal censorships cease with the analytic interpretation of the return of the repressed, or at least recede with the aid of more tolerable compromises. The censorship of the Freud-Fliess letters, the banning of the late Ferenczi, and the eradication of Emmy von N.'s memories stem from the same type of deliberate action: somebody has thrown external obstacles in the way of their eventual return to individual or collective consciousness. This is why Freud's most widely used concepts—prohibition versus desire, the superego, the Oedipus complex, instincts and their vicissitudes—fail to account for censorship and secrets in the history of the psychoanalytic movement.

What is the use of pinpointing the contradictions of psychoanalysis between its theoretical aim of openness and its institutional history of obstruction? Is it possible to bring the two extremes together? In a best-case scenario, a fictive encounter between openness and censorship could promote internal criticism within psychoanalysis. The history of psychoanalysis would then play the critical role of reader or analyst for Freudian theories, ultimately inspiring new insights. Thus the somewhat murky history of psychoanalysis—involving, among other anomalies, a case of memory eradication, a secret council, the organized ostracism of internal criticism, and the censorship of primary historical documents—could be used to extend existing theories on the problem of individual or family-based psychic secrets to the study of social groups and organizations.[4]

A final question needs to be raised. How can we explain the censorship and secrets that permeate the history of psychoanalysis from 1889 to 1957 if not beyond? Is it logical to conjecture a personal or familial secret in Freud himself? Whatever its cause or specific content may be, such a secret must be related to the basic contradiction that separates psychoanalytic theory from its history. On the one hand, Freud devised clinical and theoretical tools for the detection of psychological repression and censorship; on the other hand and often at the same time, he and his disciples created areas of inaccessible silence, thwarting all attempts at discovery.

IV

Gaining Insight into Freud

Methodological Issues

Is Freudian psychoanalysis beset by the mute pain of its creator? Did the most comprehensive investigation to date of psychic turmoil arise from suffering? Are these questions similar to asking whether Kafka and Edgar Allan Poe wrote because they suffered, whether, in giving birth to their artistic creations, they held their inner turmoil at bay? But they were writers of fiction and Freud a theoretician—of the psyche. Nevertheless, we will assert here that personal trauma constitutes the implacable if nearly imperceptible force driving Freudian contradictions. We also believe that the suffering at the root of the contrarieties of Freud's thought escaped his own theoretical and clinical instruments.

There must be some flaw in this reasoning. After all, to drown one's misery in literature is one thing, but to enmesh personal suffering in a scientific inquiry is quite another. Aren't empirical observations and theoretical claims either objectively valid or invalid, and, in any case, detached from the investigator's private circumstances? Why should the situation be any different for Freud and his psychoanalytic theories? Aren't we trying to discredit Freud's personality by this chorus of accusations? Why not be content with showing the tensions of Freud's thought without involving him personally?

We answer simply. By examining the ways in which personal or familial trauma shapes theoretical investigations, we throw light on the genesis of Freudian psychoanalysis. Indeed, unlike other investigative disciplines, psychoanalysis presupposes a close link between understanding oneself and gaining insight into others. The analytical capacity of hearing and welcoming the genuine individuality of patients is directly proportional to the degree of freedom or hindrance with which analysts can view themselves and their families. From the very beginning Freud recognized self-knowledge as a necessary condition for the psychological study of others, and accordingly, in the 1890s, he undertook his self-analysis.

To move ahead, we propose a new approach. We fall short in the search for the origin of Freudian theories if we confine our study to the history of ideas in medicine, biology, psychiatry, psychology, literature, philosophy, or sociology, if we limit our inquiry to nineteenth-century habits of mind and social attitudes. The paradoxes of Freudian psychoanalysis as a theory of psychotherapy cannot be sufficiently elucidated through Freud's intellectual biography and the degree of conservatism or enlightenment in his scientific convictions and social beliefs or practices. The contradictory development of Freudian theory does not derive its essence from historically or ethnically motivated factors—such as Freud's secular Judaism, the insidious effects of widespread anti-Semitism in Central Europe during his time, or his acquaintance with Talmudic forms of exegesis.

All of these elements are important, but, whether considered singly or as an integrated whole, they will not reach the problematic core of psychoanalysis. Surely it would be foolish to minimize the multiplicity and complexity of the historical, scientific, and cultural bases of Freudian ideas or practices at the end of the nineteenth century in Austria. It would be pointless as well to minimize the preeminent role of Freud's personal genius. To all of these long-recognized and well-researched issues we add the hypothesis of a traumatic shock suffered by Freud, a trauma that—suffused in his scientific training, his literary, philosophical, and artistic interests, his secular convictions, his ethnic background, and his social choices—underlies and sustains the singular oscillation of his psychological theories.

We want to determine to what extent Freud's person is intertwined with his theories. We seek to uncover the inner sources of his contradictory elaboration of psychoanalysis; we want to understand the psychological reasons for the paradoxical style and antagonistic forms of his thought. The following questions have guided our research:

Is it possible to pinpoint through a study of Freud's texts—without appealing to therapeutic efficacy or failure—the genuinely fruitful aspects of his thought and designate those which need to be revamped or eliminated?

In other words, what inherent methodological principles in Freud's thought allow us to distinguish between those elements of his theory which promote free inquiry and those which threaten or impede it?

Can we explain why Freudian psychoanalysis is self-contradictory, why it undermines its own effectiveness with fundamental methodological divisions?

Why did Freud found a new therapeutic discipline, one devoted to the study of the symptomatic expression of individual psychic pain, while at the same time he attempted to fix universal psychic configurations (such as penis envy, the castration complex, the death drive) that thwarted his search for the unique and unpredictable sources of individual suffering?

If a trauma did shake Freud, what was its nature and why should it have eluded the grasp of Freud's own concepts and self-analysis?

Can an inaccessible personal trauma explain the oscillating methodological thrust of his work?

Our working hypothesis is as follows. A family disaster, which occurred when Freud was nine years old, is at the root of his contradictory psychoanalytic investigations. In great part inaccessible, this trauma exercised contrary influences on Freud: it both propelled and restrained his research. Hence the internal methodological splits of psychoanalysis. We contend that Freud received the impulse for his psychoanalytic inquiries unwittingly, during his childhood and for traumatic reasons. Our position, which we will develop in the following three chapters, is this: Freud himself is the key to Freudian theoretical contradictions.

Are we here echoing the common attack that he accomplished no more than to dress in pseudo-scientific garb his own obsessions and neuroses? Definitely not. We assert something quite different. Freud's theories—whose fundamental contribution to the progress of knowledge in clinical psychology, the humanities, and the social sciences should be beyond dispute—suffered from their author's compulsory ignorance of crucial aspects of his family's life. In short, Freud conducted his psychological investigations of himself and others against the backdrop of a permanent blackout about his own traumatic history.

This situation is all the more significant because Freud's clinical and theoretical ambitions focused on the possibility of gaining access to even the most obscure regions of the psyche. Yet the darkness he met with in his own family placed him at odds with his psychological inquiries. The silence surrounding the familial drama has led to the paradoxical status of psychoanalysis. The most far-reaching attempt to understand the human psyche constantly collided with an absence and sometimes even a refusal of understanding. Our goal then is to bring to light, for Freud's sake and ours, the nature and intensity of his family's trauma—in order to free psychoanalysis from the contradictions that have plagued it since its inception and that continue to threaten it to this day despite countless attempts at improvement and renewal.

Should we lend a psychoanalytic ear to Freud? Certainly, it is crucial to address this issue if we are to resolve the question we raised earlier: What explains the epistemological impasses in which Freud became trapped? Surely, most thinkers come across insoluble problems they may acknowledge as such or not, problems they may attempt to overcome in time or not. We want to understand, in a spirit of psychoanalytic sympathy, the obstacles within Freudian thought, the obstructions that have thrown its fundamental premises into disharmony.

Thus we should like to elucidate why Freud invented a self-defeating theory of dream interpretation, providing dreamers with an unprecedented avenue to express themselves freely even as he chained them to the principle of permanent and universal meanings. Similarly we want to know why Freud framed the etiology of neurosis in a perplexing choice between truth and lies. Why did he constrain his inquiries for many a year in a quandary over factual reality and fantasized fiction? Other fundamental discrepancies have been revealed as we have surveyed Freud's work, for example the contradiction inherent in his project of "applied psychoanalysis." For the sake of applying his previously established psychoanalytic doctrine, Freud at times went so far as to diagnose nonexistent pathologies. In claiming, for instance, that a novella by the Austrian author Jensen staged the Freudian idea of sexual repression and carried out a Freudian form of psychotherapy, Freud distorted the work at hand. As a result, he also trapped the idea of dynamic sexual repression, one of his most original insights.

The contradictory theory of dream interpretation, the vacillation over the etiology of neurosis, the flawed project of applied psychoanalysis, and the institutional incongruity of openness versus censorship and secrecy in the history of the psychoanalytic movement—all exhibit a common feature. Freud merges analytic tools affording unique insight with ideas and techniques that block the progress of understanding. This methodological rift at the heart of psychoanalysis is the effect of an as yet unanalyzed traumatic division in Freud himself.

10

The Freud Family's Disaster Seen through the Original Documents

We have examined some of the major contradictions that have unsettled the theory, the practice, the literary application, and the historical transmission of psychoanalysis. Now we come to the question: Why did Freud not perceive the contradictions or feel that they were detrimental to the harmonious progress of his field of inquiry? Just as this question arose, we became aware of a set of hitherto unpublished or unexplored documents concerning the Freud family's life in 1865 and 1866. At the time, Sigmund Freud was nine and ten years old. We believe that these documents are crucial for understanding the root of Freudian contradictions. At first, we will merely print the relevant documents in the very state they reached us—that is, without commentary (the translations from the German are our own).[1]

Neue Freie Presse [New Free Press], 22 June 1865

General News. Vienna, June 21. Our correspondent F reports: For the last several days forged ruble notes have been exchanged in various banks in town of such exact likeness that only after several hundred had already been in circulation were they recognized as counterfeit. The Imperial-Royal Police succeeded yesterday in arresting the dealer.

Neue Freie Presse, 26 June 1865

Our correspondent F reports: The dealer of the counterfeit fifty ruble notes, who was arrested last week, has already made several confessions and has named several accomplices to the imperial court [of law]. Following which, and with the aid of telegraphic messages, a second dealer was arrested on the 22nd of this month in Leipzig and transferred to Vienna.

Wiener Abendpost [Vienna Evening Post], 22 February 1866

Court Proceedings:

(*Circulation of counterfeit fifty ruble notes.* Final proceedings against Josef Freud and Osias Weich for their participation in counterfeiting. Presiding judge: Mr. President of the District Jurisdiction Ritter von Schwartz. Prosecution: Mr. Motloch. Defense attorneys: Dr. Neuda and Dr. Alfred Stern.)

Having reported previously on the indictments, we now report as follows. According to his own confession, the businessman Josef Freud asked Commissioner Simon Weiss to help him find a person who might wish to buy 400 50-ruble notes; somebody wanted to sell them at a discount because they were false.

After receiving a sample for examination, witness Weiss pretended to accept the idea; he assured Freud that a buyer for the rubles was ready, and that he [Weiss] would therefore like to be able to deliver the counterfeits. However, Freud wanted to deal directly with that man; this is why Weiss, who in the meantime had notified the police about the arrangements, took Freud, on 20 June 1865, to the Hotel Victoria and introduced him to a man who indeed bought from the defendant all 400 notes of 50 rubles at 10 percent of their nominal value.

The man in question gave an additional sum of 200 florins to Weiss in payment for the ruble notes. The balance was to be paid when he had handed over the remainder of the notes.

The defendant promised to return right away and left with Weiss; but, since Freud did not want Weiss to know where he was going to fetch the rubles, Weiss had to wait for him.

Freud came back after hardly an hour. Weiss accompanied him to the same hotel where he [Freud] counted out 100 50-ruble notes for the same man; at that point he was apprehended and detained. A search of his apartment turned up an additional 259 identical ruble notes, hidden in a hat box, next to an English envelope in blue linen. All in all, Freud had 359 counterfeit ruble notes with a nominal value of 17,950 rubles.

Josef Freud, originally a businessman in Galatz, had lived for twenty years in Jassy with his family and came to Vienna in 1861 as a sales representative of the Loebl Co. of Galatz.

He alleges that he met Osias Weich as early as 1864 in Galatz and dined with him rather frequently at the Zuckermann Hotel. That is where Weich supposedly said to him: "Freud, you could make your fortune with me. I have a good deal for you." Then Weich allegedly told him that he had bought some false rubles from a man in England and that the "merchandise" had cost him 25 percent [of its actual value]; he would only like to make a little profit on it and would ask Freud no more than 5 percent commission if he sold the banknotes. At that time, however, Freud did not accept the proposition.

But following several meetings with Osias Weich here in Vienna in 1864, Freud allegedly lent him 300 florins because he was in financial trouble. Weich supposedly gave him as a security deposit, and without receiving any payment, the confiscated rubles. Eighty banknotes were supposedly stored in the confiscated English envelope.

Josef Freud traveled several times with Osias Weich to Leipzig and allegedly sent him a postal money order of 25 florins as a gift on 13 June 1865.

Freud's arraignment eventually led to Osias Weich's arrest in Leipzig on 21 June 1865, in Sophienbad. At the time of his arrest, the aforementioned had 48 thalers, and the day before had sent 25 florins to his wife in Czernowitz; in addition, he had a list of addresses of highly suspicious persons residing in England, as well as five envelopes that were very similar to the ones confiscated from Josef Freud.

Osias Weich, who could not credibly show any regular occupation, lived in London from winter to May of 1865— far away from his family—and then in Leipzig. Both after his arrest and now, he rejects amid numerous curses the accusations Freud leveled against him. He claims that he received neither a loan of 300 florins nor 25 florins as a gift from Freud; actually, he owes him [Weich] 20 florins because he paid his [Freud's] hotel bill at the Garni Hotel at the Leipzig Fair in 1864. As for counterfeit rubles, he never spoke of any, never had any, and does not even know what they look like.

According to the Russian Imperial Bank's report, the ruble notes confiscated from Josef Freud are counterfeit, were manufactured on ordinary paper, were either engraved or lithographed, and their genuine counterparts have the value of good, crisp money that is everywhere in circulation.

Given that Josef Freud intended to circulate the rubles with Weiss's help and that all the circumstances point to Osias Weich as the source of the counterfeit money, they were both convicted of participating in the distribution of counterfeit bank notes.

Wiener Zeitung [Vienna Herald], 23 February 1866

(*Distribution of counterfeit fifty ruble notes;* continued from the report in the *Wiener Abendpost* [Vienna Evening Post]):

Josef Freud, native of Tismenitz in Galicia, forty years of age, a married businessman, directly accused his codefendant Osias Weich during the proceedings of having provided him with confiscated counterfeit rubles in exchange for a loan of 300 florins. In effect, he alleges to have heard Weich say that in 1863 he [Weich] had gone to England to buy counterfeits at 25 percent of their value and that Weich had complained that it was too expensive and that he felt cheated.

Osias Weich, native of Wisnek in Bukovina, forty years of age, father of five children, allegedly a businessman, rejects Freud's accusations as slander. Background checks in Czernowitz, where his wife and children live, have shown that Osias Weich left Czernowitz by himself in the fall of 1863 and that, at that time, he still dressed as a traditional orthodox Jew. Later on, his appearance changed entirely as he began wearing German-style clothing, and, in his house, a degree of prosperity appeared that astonished everyone. This is why, on his visits to Vienna, Weich called himself Mr. Baron.

After rejecting Osias Weich's defense attorney's plea for a postponement, the state prosecutor rose to speak: "When, in far-off lands, revolutionaries cast their burning sparks toward the Continent, [sparks] that injure the emperor's prerogatives as well as those of the bourgeoisie," it is then necessary to make use of the law and give their just punishment to the criminals.

It has become equally clear that the manufacture of the 50-ruble notes occurred in England, on a much larger scale unfortunately, and that those involved in passing the counterfeits were for the most part Polish Jews.

The prosecution established in Freud's case his attempted participation in the issue of counterfeit banknotes, and required a sentence of ten years in prison for him and twelve years for Osias Weich as the instigator.

After the closing arguments by the defense, the rebuttal by the prosecution, and the answer by the defense, the court announced, following a relatively lengthy period of deliberation, this judgment:

Josef Freud and Osias Weich are both guilty of the crime of aiding and abetting the issue of counterfeit banknotes; they will both be condemned to a prison sentence of ten years' duration.

In Josef Freud's case, numerous attenuating circumstances will prompt the court to submit the papers to the Supreme Court for an extraordinary easing of the penalty.

Both defendants declared their intention to appeal.

Neue Freie Presse, 23 February 1866

Court Proceedings:

Vienna, 22 February 1866. (Counterfeit Affair) Presiding judge: Ritter von Schwartz. State prosecutor: Mr. Motloch. Defense lawyers: Dr. Neuda and Dr. Alfred Stern.

The accused are Josef Freud, born in Tismenitz (Galicia), forty years old, tradesman, and Osias Weich, born in Wisnek (Bukovina), forty years old, tradesman. In the indictment, drawn up by the state prosecutor, the following facts appear. In May 1865 Josef Freud asked Commissioner Simon Weiss to help him find a buyer for 100 50-ruble notes; someone intended to sell them cheaply because they were counterfeits. Weiss pretended to accept the offer, asked for a sample counterfeit bill, and then left, ostensibly to find a buyer. In possession of the counterfeit note, he went to the police. He later arranged a meeting with Josef Freud at the Victoria Hotel and proceeded to buy 400 of the 50-ruble notes, for which he gave a down payment of 200 florins. The balance was to be paid when the remainder of the merchandise (the counterfeit currency) was handed over, but when Weiss came to collect it, and Freud had the counterfeit currency with him, the latter was apprehended by the security forces.

He was carrying 100 counterfeit notes; a search of his apartment turned up an additional 259. According to Freud's deposition he had met Osias Weich in Galatz during the summer of 1864. The two of them used to dine together quite often in the Zuckermann Hotel. One day Weich asked him [Freud] whether he would like to make some money, adding that he [Weich] had purchased some counterfeit rubles from an Englishwoman at 25 percent of their face value; Weich would be willing to sell them at a commission of only 5 percent; all Freud would have to do would be to pass them. Freud allegedly refused this proposition. He claims that in September 1864 Weich had come to Vienna, met with him at the Café Wagner in Leopoldstadt, and asked him to lend him 300 florins. Freud alleges that he lent him the 300 florins and received, in an English envelope, the confiscated forgeries as a security deposit. He [Freud] went on to claim that he had met Weich repeatedly at the Fair in Leipzig, and since Weich continued to be badly off, sent him 25 florins by mail order. Following this deposition, Weich was looked for, located in Leipzig, arrested, and subsequently transferred to Vienna. Weich, who could not credibly show that he had any profession, carried with him a list of addresses in London of persons who are regarded as highly suspect. According to information available to the court through diplomatic channels, they included the name of Mrs. Levy, a Jewish woman known for passing fraudulent currency. In addition, he was carrying several envelopes of the exact same shape and size as the one in which Freud kept his rubles, and thus fashioned in a way as to fit 50-ruble bills. According to the Russian Imperial Bank's report from St. Petersburg, the notes found in Josef Freud's possession were produced by copper engraving and lithographic print on ordinary paper. They are the same as the other counterfeit notes that have been swamping European financial institutions and that have already led to numerous criminal convictions. Another report from Leipzig leads one to suspect that Osias Weich is the same person who, several years ago and in Polish disguise, bought several watches from Swiss watchmakers at Leipzig, paying with counterfeit notes that were quite similar to the ones in our matter.

The defense used by the accused was at times extremely violent. During the final proceedings, just as during the preliminary inquest, Freud volunteered confessions and accused Weich of having given him the counterfeit notes as a deposit. Extraordinarily irritated, Weich rejected all these accusations as untrue, claiming that Freud, whose family lives in London, was using him so as to be able to designate someone as the provider of the counterfeit money. His [Freud's] assertions [Weich continued] might indeed seem plausible since the two of them had traveled together, a fact that Freud must have shrewdly contrived. Yet, the whole thing is nothing but a tissue of lies. Weich alleged that he possessed the addresses from London because, as is quite possible, he found them in a hotel room and took them, a thing easily done when traveling. Weich justified his having the English envelopes, which were similar to the ones in which Freud kept his counterfeits, with the allegation that Freud often used his, Weich's, suitcase when traveling, and therefore the envelopes had simply been left in the suitcase. The accused continued to blame and to insult each other, but did not succeed in shaking the validity of the indictment. The prosecutor asked for ten years in prison for Freud and twelve years for Weich, both without probation.

The court rendered its verdict in the late afternoon. "Josef Freud and Osias Weich are found guilty of aiding and abetting the issue of counterfeit bank notes; for which reason they will be imprisoned for a term of ten years." The court resolved to hand over Freud's case to the Supreme Court with a view to seeking terms of leniency.

The condemned announced their intention to appeal.

*Austrian Police Minister Belcredi's Memorandum
to Count Mensdorff, Foreign Secretary,
16 October 1865*

A third case of attempted distribution of counterfeit ruble notes was uncovered in Vienna. On 20 June the Israelite

Josef Freud was apprehended as he was about to sell 100 counterfeit bills, with a nominal value of 17,950 rubles. According to his deposition, Josef Freud is Jewish, married, and the father of two children; he was born in Tismenitz, in the district of Stanislau in Galicia; however, he spent most of his life in Moldavia. He married in 1849 in Jassy and later had a business selling English hardware. Since 1861 he has been living in Vienna, and has since then made three trips to London, Manchester, and Birmingham, and has also visited Leipzig, Breslau, etc., and has had frequent correspondence with foreign countries. His son-in-law, Adolf Kornhauser, living in Trencsin in Hungary and suspected of being an accomplice to Freud, has been arrested. About the bank notes Freud knew were counterfeits, he stated during his deposition that he obtained them from someone named Osias Weich, native of Czernowitz, whose acquaintance he had allegedly made in Galatz last year, during the latter's stay in Vienna.

Following an inquiry, it appeared that Osias Weich had stayed in Vienna on several occasions, for example between 11 and 13 April of last year, the period during which Leo Krongold, of whom I spoke earlier [in a portion of the memorandum not reproduced here], had also been there.

Like the others, this third case leads one to believe that the real source of the counterfeit money is in England. This seems to be borne out by two highly suspicious letters sent from England by two sons, currently living in Manchester, of a brother of Josef Freud's. In one of these letters we are told that the brother's sons have as much money as there is sand by the sea and that, since they are being wise, clever, and circumspect, fortune will not fail to smile on them. In another letter, they ask him whether the good star of the Freud house has risen for him as well; they go on to ask him to find a bank for the merchandise where the turnover would be larger, faster, and more profitable. (Translated from the German transcription in Gicklhorn, *Sigmund Freud und der Onkeltraum,* 39–40)

These documents can also be found in the Freud Archives of the Library of Congress in Washington, D.C. The updated catalog (1990) of the Sigmund Freud Collection classifies them under the following headings: "Totally Restricted Files Z4 Year 2000. Family Papers: Freud, Josef: photocopies and microfilms of documents regarding conviction for counterfeiting rubles."

These documents about Sigmund Freud's uncle Josef interest us because we believe they can help us locate the source of the theoretical, clinical, and institutional contradictions in Freudian psychoanalysis.

Freud's Self-Analysis and the Field of Biographical Studies

We have asked: What was the trauma that upset Freud's family, and why did it escape Freud's self-analysis? Before attempting to give an answer, with the help of the documents we are publishing here, we will find it useful to consider Freud's self-analysis and some of the biographical or conceptual research that has grown up around it.

As is well known, Freud undertook his self-analysis in October 1896 at the latest, after his father's death. Some scholars have called Freud's self-analysis a unique and extraordinary event in western thought because, they say, it led to the discovery of psychoanalysis itself. Why suppose, then, that a self-analysis might have been insufficient to reveal Freud to himself? Let us recall that his self-analysis, so very useful for deepening Freud's clinical intuitions, did have its stumbling blocks. We can hear Freud say so to his friend Fliess on 14 November 1897: "My self-analysis remains interrupted. I have realized why I can analyze myself only with the help of knowledge acquired objectively (like an outsider).

True self-analysis is impossible; otherwise there would be no [neurotic] illness. Since I am still contending with some kind of puzzle in my patients, this is bound to hold me up in my own analysis as well" (CL, 281).

According to many authors of various stripes, Freud shifted his theoretical paradigm fundamentally as a result of his self-analysis in 1897: he replaced forever his theory of traumatic seduction in childhood with the theory of sexually grounded fantasies of seduction. On this point we disagree with these other scholars. Basing our assessment on the many contradictory statements in Freud's letters and writings (see Chapter 2), we doubt very much that Freud's self-analysis did truly usher in the harmonious discovery of psychoanalysis. Instead, the evidence overwhelmingly suggests that the years of self-analysis coincided with a period of intense theoretical vacillation.

We will go further. Our study of Freud's letters and works forces us to question whether a clean theoretical break ever occurred, either in 1897 or at any time afterward. This is why we choose to highlight the vicissitudes of Freud's struggle: one of his positions seems to gain the upper hand at any one time, only to be upset in short order by the other. The new position, apparently growing stronger by the day, unexpectedly totters under the weight of Freud's periodic return to his former position. Only many years after 1897 could Freud say with a cool head that he had at that time definitively rejected his seduction theory. We have shown that even as he was confirming in 1915 (in *The History of the Psycho-Analytic Movement*) the irrevocable replacement of his "erroneous" theory of infantile seduction, he was about to write or publish his case study of the Wolf Man and the twenty-third of his *Introductory Lectures on Psycho-Analysis*, both of which display his theoretical fluctuations.

We are in a position, therefore, to corroborate Freud's momentary evaluation of 14 November 1897: the mystery that continued to puzzle him in his clinical work was enough to stop his self-analysis. The only difference is that we are extending this evaluation to the whole of Freud's self-analytical period (1897–1900), if not well beyond. We contend that Freud's persistent theoretical vacillation about the importance of real versus fantasized seductions robbed him of the certainty that he could ever obtain objective or verifiable clinical knowledge. It was as though the precondition of self-analysis—defined by Freud as a mirror-like reflection between understanding oneself and understanding others—simply could not be fulfilled in his case. Assailed by doubts as to whether he really understood his patients, could he hope to analyze himself serenely and without further ado?

For many years scholars have praised the value of Freud's analysis by Freud. To study its unfolding, they have used Freud's accounts in *The Interpretation of Dreams* (1900) and *The Psychopathology of Everyday Life* (1901), and his letters to Fliess (1887–1904). Didier Anzieu, Edith Buxbaum, Ernst Kris, and others have established links between Freud's self-analysis and his theoretical development.[2] Thus Anzieu created a parallel between Freud's dreams, screen memories, and daydreams and his discovery of basic psychoanalytic concepts, such as castration anxiety, incestuous wishes, unconscious fantasies, the Oedipus complex, the family romance, infantile sexuality, primal scenes, the dreamwork, and the forgetting of proper names. Anzieu sees an exact correspondence between Freud's self-analysis and the systematic development of his psychoanalytic arsenal. Consequently, Anzieu concludes his study by stating that, in his self-analysis, Freud's principal aim was not so much understanding himself as gaining general knowledge about the psychological structure of the normal human mind.

We could not agree more, save for one reservation. Given Freud's concurrent vacillation about the causes of neurosis (traumatic seduction versus infantile sexuality), we wonder whether his self-analysis could have provided him with reliable insights into the human mind in general. Faced with doubts—Are my patients lying to me? Am I being led down the wrong theoretical path?—Freud's attempt to turn to himself for a trustworthy model of the human mind is quite understandable. This endeavor at the dawn of the twentieth century seems to us exceptional as well; it is comparable perhaps, in its breadth and poignant humanity, to the *Confessions* of Rousseau or Saint Augustine. Still, the attempt at self-analysis failed to free Freud's thought from the theoretical oscillation he might have hoped to resolve.

Another group of scholars, in particular Wladimir Granoff, Alexander Grinstein, and Conrad Stein, treat Freud's self-analysis with a view to enriching Freud's own associative material.[3] They complete Freud's associations to his dreams by drawing upon and collating a large number of his texts (whether self-analytical or not), his symptoms (reported by himself, his disciples, or his biographers), events and sundry anecdotes from his life, his favorite books, words, phrases, or jokes (essentially Jewish humor). Through the efforts of these scholars we can indeed gain valuable insight into Freud's dreams, for example through the detailed summary of the literary works he mentioned in passing in his associations, or through the precise identification of the real-life persons who appear disguised in his dreams. In short, these authors expand or create networks of association in order to propose unconscious motives for specific self-analytical issues, often indicated by Freud himself, such as his long-lasting inability to visit Rome. In addition, the initial publication of the Freud-Fliess letters in 1950 aroused a great deal of critical interest in the unconscious aspects of Freud's relationship to his friend. Such studies are eminently successful when it comes to subjecting Freud the man to a strictly Freudian kind of psychological inquiry. All of the above-mentioned scholars and their many followers have attempted to make sense of Freud's life by using the analytical tools invented by Freud himself.

Our research places us in a distinctly different position. We have conjectured a trauma at the root of Freud's investigations, a type of trauma that never received explicit theoretical attention in his work. It seems to us, furthermore, that the young Freud's family disaster is the blind spot of the adult's thought; this is so because his thought excludes its own secret point of origin. As a result it is impossible to analyze Freud the man with Freudian instruments. Of course, it would be pointless to insist that one could not clear up this or that aspect of Freud's internal life with the help of his own ideas. Without wanting to slight anyone, Freud or his disciples, we are convinced nevertheless of the inadequacy of Freudian ideas when it comes to assessing the fundamental upheaval that threw Freud as well as his theory into disharmony.

For years we have been leaning toward the following hypothesis: the nature of the family disaster bewildering Freud in his childhood was such that his self-analysis could not have explored it. This idea connects us with the methodological shift that Max Schur (Freud's personal physician during his final years) introduced in Freudian biographical studies when, in 1966, he published his article "Some Additional 'Day Residues' of the 'Specimen Dream of Psychoanalysis.'"[4] In this ground-breaking essay Schur showed that Freud's model dream in *The Interpretation of Dreams* rests on biographical and professional facts that Freud deliberately did not divulge. Schur carried the dream analysis further than Freud by using unpublished sources and by bringing to bear on the dream relevant information that Freud gave elsewhere. Schur later intensified this line of questioning in his book *Freud: Living and Dying* (1972).

Basing his work on what he supposed were recently discovered documents, Schur surmised that Freud's father, Jakob, married three times rather than twice (as had been the common belief until then) and that the woman he allegedly married second bore the name Rebecca. The family supposedly hid her existence and the circumstances of her subsequent disappearance from Sigmund Freud, the eldest son born to Jakob's next wife. With this supposition Schur initiated a speculative line of research founded on an alleged distance between the Freud family's "fictions" and the "truth" revealed by the documents. In this connection Schur advocated the study of the traces the father's hidden second wife and her death might have left in Freud's self-analytical remarks and/or theories.

Though we are skeptical about the trustworthiness of the documents Schur invoked (and in this we are not alone; see Marianne Krüll, *Freud and His Father*), we recognize the novelty of Schur's approach. He was the first scholar to conjecture that a potential "secret" in the father's life might have found its way into the son's theoretical works. In short, even though our incredulity is boundless when it comes to the content of Schur's speculation—that a rejected and concealed second wife of Jakob Freud's might have died of sorrow—we do resonate with the crux of Schur's question: To what extent did his family's life influence Freud's theories?

The late 1970s constituted a crucial period in Freud studies; new voices, some inspired by Schur, others not, increasingly began raising the question of the interrelation between Freud's family and his theories. Marie Balmary, Marianne Krüll, Barbro Sylwan, and Maria Torok are the main representatives of this trend. Concurrently, though in very different ways, they attempted to reach into the unanalyzed portions of Freud's mind.

Marie Balmary draws directly on Schur's speculative hypothesis; elaborating on it, she hopes to ground it. In her book *Psychoanalyzing Psychoanalysis: The Hidden Fault of the Father* (1979; English translation 1982), Jakob Freud's secret, a repudiated and dead Rebecca (possibly driven into suicide), forces a dramatic entry into his son's psychological theories. According to Balmary, Freud repudiated his early seduction theory for purely personal reasons, because the seduction theory amounted to a theory of sexual mistakes committed by adults. Now, Freud's self-analysis might have unconsciously revealed to him his own father's hidden fault or sin; to avoid seeing that, Freud allegedly preferred to replace the theory of adult perversion (the seduction theory) with a theory in which the burden of sexual perversion is shifted onto the child (the Oedipus complex). Balmary sees Freud's shift in 1897 as a desperate attempt to invent a sin for the son in order to erase the "sin of the father." In short, for Balmary, the Oedipus complex (the son's complex) is a barrier or defense against the personal and possibly universal truth of Freud's initial discovery about his elders' sins.

Marianne Krüll published her book in 1979 as well. In the French edition of 1983, she pointed out the similarity of her views with Balmary's. True, the basic question is the same, though the road leading to it and the answers are quite different. Both authors accept the idea that Freud shifted his theoretical direction irrevocably in 1897; both turn this shift into a psychological symptom somehow having to do with Freud's father. The difference is that for Balmary the issue is the influence of a father's hidden sins on his son, whereas Krüll is interested in Freud's father's guilt about sexuality in general and in his departures from his ancestors' conservative religious and moral tenets. In these differing ways, then, both Balmary and Krüll conclude that Freud revoked his early seduction theory because in his new theory of infantile sexuality he found an effective means to repress his own father's hidden life and/or guilt.

The originality of Krüll's approach stems from her historical research into the life of orthodox Jews in Austria-Hungary during Freud's father's lifetime. This allows her to offer insight into the probable emotional repercussions of the desire to become an assimilated Jew. She also conjectures the insidious influence of a father's social, religious, and sexual taboos on his son's development. As a result, she asks about the role of silence in a family's life. What is it like for a child when his parents forbid him to know of their inhibitions or transgressions? Krüll's answer is that the children become just like the adults.

For example, Freud exerted his father's own inhibiting influence on his disciples. Several of his works and theories, especially *Totem and Taboo* (1910) and *Moses and Monotheism* (1938) bear the mark of his father's reticence about himself:

> Freud's theories should not be accepted unreservedly; they must be tested carefully with a view to determining which of them merely served Freud to disguise important problems that impinged on Jacob's taboo. Such theories certainly include the myth of primal patricide based on the belief in phylogenetic inheritance, and hence, ultimately, the entire Oedipus theory and all concepts and constructs based upon it. These are mystifications that obscure the interhuman dimension, ignoring the role of the social environment in the socialization of man, and hence its role in the emergence of "normal" or of socially deviant behavior. They have led psychoanalysis, in theory and therapeutic practice, into a blind alley.   (Krüll, *Freud and His Father,* 212)

Unlike Balmary, who upholds the preeminence of Freud's early seduction theory, Krüll proposes a non-Freudian theoretical model, the interpersonal and family-oriented dimension, to help us understand Freud and to enrich psychoanalytic theory as a whole.

We recognize the value of these investigations, though our research into Freud has caused us to ask different questions and to propose different answers. We agree only in principle with Balmary's attempt to flesh out Schur's hypothesis that hitherto unsuspected factors in the Freud family's life might have affected Freud's theories. As for Krüll, we feel a methodological affinity with her combination of historical, sociological, and psychoanalytic approaches. However, we categorically reject the presupposition that underlies both studies. We see no evidence that Freud definitively shifted his theoretical paradigm in 1897 (see Parts I and III). Thus we cannot agree with either Balmary's or Krüll's contention that Freud's subsequent theories acted as an unconsciously erected bulwark against realizing his father's guilt. We believe that Freud's views never underwent a single or simple conversion, but that his theories moved through cycles of oscillation and disruption, cycles in which contradictions were perpetually created, calmed for a time, and yet inexorably renewed.

This is why we offer our historical and psychoanalytic hypothesis of a family trauma that shook Freud's childhood. It was a trauma whose essential features remained obscure for the child, producing doubts, suspicions, and contradictions in the adult's theories. Consequently, we do not believe that any particular theory by Freud (such as the Oedipus complex or phylogenetic inheritance) ever disguised his personal problems. Instead, his unwittingly endured family trauma upset his methods of research, inhibiting or stopping the possibility of free inquiry. Rather than criticize discrete ideas by Freud, we propose to view the whole of his enterprise as a thwarted theory of psychological investigation. His family's silence provoked an investigative blockage in Freud.

Also in the late 1970s but quite independently from Schur, Balmary, or Krüll, Maria Torok became acquainted with new biographical documents (published in part by Renée Gicklhorn in *Sigmund Freud und der Onkeltraum* [Sigmund Freud and the Uncle Dream], 1976). These documents gave Torok an unexpected basis for pursuing a casual suggestion by Nicolas Abraham that a family secret (perhaps similar to the Wolf Man's) might have played a role in Freud's theories. The new biographical data about Freud's uncle Josef were of particular interest to Torok, as she had studied, in collaboration with Abraham, the unintended transmission of family secrets and had demonstrated their paramount importance for a general psychological understanding of individuals and groups as well as for psychotherapy.[5] Her research on Freud resulted initially in a programmatic article, followed by a series of other articles, all of which offered the idea that numerous instances of Freud's clinical blindness were symptomatic of his family's secret and traumatic past.[6]

Freud's Dreams:
Witnesses to His Family Disaster

A disaster struck the Freud family in 1865 when Sigmund Freud was nine years old. On 20 June 1865, acting on an informant's lead, the police arrested his uncle Josef Freud for selling counterfeit rubles. Sentenced in a public trial to ten years' imprisonment, he served it in harsh conditions that included weekly days of fasting. He gained his release after a few years, probably through an appeal filed by his relatives.

Josef Freud's case was part of a larger counterfeiting scandal encompassing several European countries, including Germany, England, Austria-Hungary, France, Poland, and Russia. Trials of counterfeiters had taken place ever since 1863, but starting in 1865 extensive diplomatic and police efforts established the existence of a network whose headquarters were presumably in England. Contemporary Austrian newspapers published detailed reports of the arrests, court proceedings, and prison sentences of the various counterfeiters, among them Josef Freud (see Chapter 10). In a confidential memorandum the Austrian police minister quoted two letters written to Josef Freud by his nephews Philip and Emmanuel, Sigmund Freud's half-brothers; because of these letters, the minister suspected that the forged notes were manufactured in England. The minister urged, in vain as it turned out, that further judicial inquiries be made there. Here is the crucial excerpt from the memorandum:

> Like the others, this third case [the case of Josef Freud] leads one to believe that the real source of the counterfeit money is in England. This seems borne out by two highly suspicious letters sent from England by two sons, currently residing in Manchester, of a brother of Josef Freud's. In one of these letters we are told that the brother's sons have as much money as there is sand by the sea and that, since they are being wise, clever, and circumspect, fortune will not fail to smile on them. In another letter, they ask him whether the good star of the Freud house has risen for him as well; they go on to ask him to find a bank for the merchandise where the turnover would be larger, faster, and more profitable.
>
> (Gicklhorn, *Sigmund Freud und der Onkeltraum*, 40)

For lack of further international collaboration, police investigators never discovered the precise place where the forgeries originated. As a result, Sigmund Freud's half-brothers (his father's sons from a first marriage) never became subject to any police action. Therefore the Austrian police minister's suspicions have never been either confirmed or denied. The only thing we can safely suppose is that Sigmund Freud's parents heard—from Josef himself, his wife, or their lawyer, before or after the arrest—of the existence and the contents of the two letters confiscated from Josef by the police.

These are the facts as based on the available documents. In themselves, they are not much. But what an upheaval in the life of a family! For the courts the matter is settled quickly: a criminal has been caught, tried, and sentenced. The social order has been reestablished. For the family, however, the emotional calamity is just beginning. They will have to face the shame, justifying themselves as best as they can to neighbors, acquaintances, and shopkeepers. No doubt everyone has read the newspapers that have besmirched the name Freud. An even greater problem arises: How to talk about the disgrace to the children in the family? Will they condemn the adults like everyone else? Will they understand that it was nothing more than a misstep, brought on perhaps by poverty or apprehension about an uncertain future in an anti-Semitic part of the world where Jews still often had the precarious existence of outcasts? How to keep or recover the child's confidence in the moral integrity of the family unit? And then, can you really tell everything to a nine-year-old (even one as precocious as the young Sigmund); can you appeal to his compassion?

Unfortunately, these types of questions, which seem eminently reasonable, tolerant, and finely attuned to the sensitive souls of children, are probably never contemplated, let alone raised. There are several ways for adults to deal with dishonorable family disasters, such as criminal behavior, shameful illnesses, suicide, madness—but they rarely if ever presuppose a young child's capacity to understand. Adults tend to give a partial or incomplete account of the events, in an attempt to discourage questions that might prove all too painful in a time of hardship. Or parents quite simply resort to lying because they feel ashamed in front of their own children.

Most often an uneasy silence reigns. The adults abruptly stop in midsentence when the child enters the room. They change the topic or ask trivial questions. Somebody tells a joke—whatever it takes to distract attention, to stifle the children's questions. It is no use: embarrassment never escapes children's emotional sagacity. The family pretends to behave as if nothing at all is the matter, as if the disaster has not even occurred, or as if it has had no effect whatsoever on the life of the family or the children's future. Still, it is usually the children who suffer most from deceit and secretiveness. Because of the many mixed signals they receive from their family, they become confused to the point of not being able to discriminate between truth and falsehood, especially if the adults are stubbornly silent and dissembling by turns.

When the family experiences the catastrophe as a stigma, free communication either with the outside world or within the family becomes practically impossible. It is quite a different matter when a natural disaster strikes a house, a village, or a region. Everybody talks about it days on end. The whole community is involved, and everyone wants to hear everything, even the most insignificant details. People help one another; they bury the dead and rescue the living. Nothing of the kind happens in the case of discredited families. Such a family feels socially isolated, sometimes even ostracized. Many family members hold on for a lifetime to a particular aspect of the traumatic event, and yet no opportunity ever presents itself for them to say what they experienced, felt, or suffered. Tears are held back; emotions congeal and are finally extinguished. Being unable to discuss the upsetting events in detail, unable to express the wounds opened in their hearts, they cannot pity themselves, cannot grieve over their own bewilderment and sorrow. Victims of the grownups' despair and haphazard dissembling, children are even less able to weep over their fate. They live in an oppressive atmosphere of silence, with the mute pain of being unable to grasp what it is they suffer from. Children raised with family secrets lack the knowledge that they are trapped by the silence of their elders.

Here we will approach Sigmund Freud's calamitous childhood as it appears to us through his own dreams. We suppose that he could never speak openly with his relatives about the traumatic effects of what had occurred, that he could not get any real answers to his questions, even if he dared to raise them. There are, of course, types of traumas or misfortunes about which one can talk freely, for example the death of a sibling or a grandmother, a car accident, an illness, the loss of livelihood, destitution. These misfortunes can be more or less easily absorbed into a family's topography because talking about them is not forbidden.[7] However, a dishonor, a stain on the family's reputation, leaves behind a permanent silence and malaise.

In our opinion, his family's silence had far-reaching repercussions on Freud's subsequent psychological inquiries. Unspeakable family traumas may have and probably did indeed propel his research, but they also obstructed it, thwarting his desire to understand individual forms of suffering. We hypothesize that Freud's family disaster is at the root of the contradictions of his thought, clinical work, and institutional practices. This is so because, due to the grave and unresolved suspicions that hung over his half-brothers, Freud's family almost certainly never allowed him to gain anything more than partial insight into crucial aspects of the trauma. It is likely that the family, not wanting to broach the subject publicly, wondered in secret for years whether Sigmund's half-brothers might eventually face arrest. (It is important to recall here the Austrian police minister's memorandum and the accusations that Osias Weich, Josef Freud's codefendant, leveled against the latter's nephews during Josef's trial in Vienna.)

In time the entire family must have learned of the two letters incriminating Sigmund's half-brothers. The whole family—except the children, of course. We are well aware that, in the years 1865–1866, Freud was no longer a little boy; being already nine or ten and precocious, he could in principle have mustered the psychological resources to deal with the shock of his uncle's arrest and imprisonment. Yet those resources were most likely wanting, as Freud's dreams will show, because other equally important elements of the drama, apart from the uncle's public trial, were kept from the child. As a result, his family's stifled anguish must have afflicted him all the more as he was not supposed to discover what it was about. The genuine trauma consisted, then, in the young Freud's inability to break through the wall of silence, to lift the veil from the family's secret. The presence of a secret disturbs the very ability to deal with a family trauma because it makes it difficult if not impossible to communicate freely even about those aspects of the disaster which are fully acknowledged by all.

No account of the Freud family's calamity has reached us from Josef, Jakob, or Sigmund Freud. However, we do have the indirect testimony of Freud's dreams as they exist in *The Interpretation of Dreams*. They allow us to put our finger on the painful effects of the family catastrophe. For example, we read in the Dream of the Uncle (of which we will say more later) that Freud's father's hair turned gray as a token of the shock. But apart from the Dream of the Uncle, in which he speaks of Josef's "crime," Freud's dreams are less than explicit concerning the impact of this "crime" on his family or himself. Hence the usefulness of deciphering the dreams, of capturing the mark of hidden suffering, and of seeing in them a constant attempt to repair the family's wounded self-image. Indeed, almost without exception, Freud's dreams keep expressing his obstinate will to succeed, his personal pride, his sense of superiority in relation to his colleagues, his thirst for grandeur and glory. Let us not be misled! This is more than a self-aware genius seeking legitimate recognition. Freud's thirst for grandeur appears side by side with the uncle's crime and the vain hope of getting rid of one's distressing ancestors. It is also significant that the one dream whose subject matter is, according to Freud, his self-analysis happens to be a nightmare. We think therefore that the bulk of Freud's dreaming, as reported in *The Interpretation of Dreams,* is designed to annul his family's nightmarish dishonor through his own striking professional success.

Here, briefly, is our methodology. We will study the following dreams: the Dream of the Uncle, Count Thun, *Non vixit,* Riding on a Horse, Open-air Closet, Botanical Monograph, and Self-dissection. We will analyze them both autonomously and as a group, as though they provided free associations for one another. We conjecture that these dreams are pieces of one complex puzzle, dispersed fragments of a crucial problem in Freud's family and his emotional life. We will listen carefully to German, the language in which Freud wrote down his dreams. And, above all, we will bear in mind the biographical documents, newspaper articles, and police reports that relate the events and suspicions surrounding Uncle Josef's arrest in 1865 for passing counterfeit rubles. Knowing about these events and suspicions in detail opens a new source for understanding Freud's dreams. Without the documents his dreams might have remained nearly silent. They would have been unable to reveal their uppermost (though most deeply hidden) concern, Josef's and the entire Freud family's traumatic history.

Having access to the documents provides us with a precise vocabulary, something akin to a concealed glossary of the counterfeiting affair, a vocabulary that can help us decipher specific elements in Freud's dreams. For example, it is not unimportant to know that, in German, a person selling forged money is called a *Verbreiter* (literally, a disseminator or someone who spreads). Fragments of this word appear disguised in Freud's dream of Riding on a Horse. In it he tells us how he put a poultice on a painful boil. If in the German word that Freud uses for boil (*Furunkel*), we hear the *uncle,* in another series of German words, involving *horse, poultice, he is riding,* we can hear fragments of the German word for *passing forged notes* (horse = *Pferd;* poultice = *Brei(umschlag);* he is riding = *reitet; f(v)erbreitet* = he sells counterfeit money). In summary, we use the new documents and their principal terms as an associative basis, as a sort of glue that lends cohesion to Freud's dreams. Together they display a bundle of ruminations, worries, and anxieties, as well as attempts, successful and unsuccessful by turns, to keep the family trauma at arm's length.

Freud often says things like this in *The Interpretation of Dreams:*

> I shall . . . only report the first half of the dream here, since the other half has no connection with the purpose for which I am describing the dream. (137)

> For reasons with which we are not concerned, I shall not pursue the interpretation of this dream any further, but will merely indicate the direction in which it lay. (173)

> Anyone who has formed even the slightest idea of the extent of condensation in dreams will easily imagine what a number of pages would be filled by a full analysis of this dream. Fortunately, however, in the present context I need only take up one point in it. (453)

Given these and similar reticences, we cannot know with certainty what meaning Freud's dreams would have had, had he given their full text or had he pursued their analysis to the end. We can only work with the elements as given, and we consider it useless to speculate on the direction his interpretations might have taken. We are convinced nevertheless that Freud would not have discussed the counterfeiting affair any more explicitly than he does in his Dream of the Uncle. The lack of emotion there shows how far removed from himself Freud would like to see the events of 1865–1866.

We do not intend to analyze all of his dreams, only a number of those that in our estimation concern his family problems. We will present excerpts from Freud's dreams and his own interpretations. We draw on James Strachey's edition of *The Interpretation of Dreams* and standard editions of the original German text. In dating the dreams, we rely on Freud's own indications and on references in the Freud-Fliess correspondence, or we use Didier Anzieu's *Freud's Self-Analysis and His Discovery of Psychoanalysis* and Alexander Grinstein's *On Sigmund Freud's Dreams*.

Dream of the Uncle

Date: Spring 1897

I. . . *My friend R. was my uncle.—I had a great feeling of affection for him.*

II. *I saw before me his face, somewhat changed. It was as though it had been drawn out lengthways. A yellow beard that surrounded it stood out especially clearly.* (I, 137–138)

Excerpts from Freud's associations and interpretation:

In the spring of 1897 I learnt that two professors at our university had recommended me for appointment as *professor extraordinarius*. [Roughly equivalent to an Assistant Professor. All such appointments in Austria were made by the Minister of Education.—Strachey's note] The news surprised and greatly delighted me since it implied recognition . . . But I at once warned myself . . . During the last few years the Ministry had disregarded recommendations of this sort . . .

One evening I had a visit from a friend . . . For a considerable time he had been a candidate for promotion to a professorship . . . He told me that . . . he had driven the exalted official [the Minister of Education] into a corner and had asked him straight out whether the delay over his appointment was not in fact due to denominational considera-

tions . . . The same denominational considerations applied
to my own case.   (I, 136–137)

"R. was my uncle." What could that mean? I never had more
than one uncle—Uncle Josef. There was an unhappy story
attached to him. Once—more than thirty years ago—in his
eagerness to make money, he allowed himself to be involved
in a transaction of a kind that is severely punished by the
law, and he was in fact punished for it. My father, whose hair
turned grey from grief in a few days, used always to say that
Uncle Josef was not a bad man but only a simpleton; those
were his words. So that if my friend R. was my Uncle Josef,
what I was meaning to say was that R. was a simpleton.
                                                    (I, 138)

I still had no idea at all what could be the purpose of this
comparison, against which I continued to struggle. It did
not go very deep, after all, since my uncle was a criminal,
whereas my friend R. bore an unblemished character . . . At
this point I remembered another conversation which I had
had a few days earlier with another colleague, N., and, now
I came to think of it, upon the same subject. I had met N.
in the street. He too had been recommended for a professorship . . . I had said . . . "you know what such a recom-
mendation is worth from your own experience." "Who can
say?" he had answered—jokingly, it seemed; "there was
something definite against *me*. Don't you know that a
woman once started legal proceedings against me? I needn't
assure you that the case was dismissed. It was a disgraceful
attempt at blackmail . . . But perhaps they may be using this
at the Ministry as an excuse for not appointing me. But *you*
have an unblemished character." This told me who the
criminal was, and at the same time showed me how the
dream was to be interpreted and what its purpose was. My

Uncle Josef represented my two colleagues who had not been appointed to professorships—the one as a simpleton and the other as a criminal. I now saw too why they were represented in this light. If the appointment of my friends R. and N. had been postponed for "denominational" reasons, my own appointment was also open to doubt; if, however, I could attribute the rejection of my two friends to other reasons, which did not apply to me, my hopes would remain untouched . . . I could rejoice at my appointment to a professorship. (I, 139–140)

What, then, could have been the origin of the ambitiousness which produced the dream in me? At that point I recalled an anecdote I had often heard repeated in my childhood. At the time of my birth an old peasant-woman had prophesied to my proud mother that with her first-born child she had brought a great man into the world . . . Could this have been the source of my thirst for grandeur? But that reminded me of another experience, dating from my later childhood, which provided a still better explanation. My parents had been in the habit, when I was a boy of eleven or twelve, of taking me with them to the Prater. One evening, while we were sitting in a restaurant there, our attention had been attracted by a man who was moving from one table to another . . . and he had been inspired to declare that I should probably grow up to be a Cabinet Minister . . . But now to return to my dream. It began to dawn on me that my dream had carried me back from the dreary present to . . . cheerful hopes . . . and that the wish that it had done its best to fulfil was one dating back to those times. In mishandling my two learned and eminent colleagues because they were Jews, and in treating the one as a simpleton and the other as a criminal, I was behaving as though

I were the Minister, I had put myself in the Minister's place. Turning the tables on His Excellency with a vengeance! He had refused to appoint me *professor extraordinarius* and I had retaliated in the dream by stepping into his shoes.

(I, 192–193)

I then recalled that there still was a piece of the dream which the interpretation had not touched. After the idea had occurred to me that R. was my uncle, I had had a warm feeling of affection for him in the dream. Where did that feeling belong? I had naturally never had any feeling of affection for my Uncle Josef. I had been fond of my friend R. and had esteemed him for many years; but if I had gone up to him and expressed my sentiments in terms approaching the degree of affection I had felt in the dream, there could be no doubt that he would have been astonished. My affection for him struck me as ungenuine and exaggerated . . . The affection in the dream did not belong to the latent content, to the thoughts that lay behind the dream; it stood in contradiction to them and was calculated to conceal the true interpretation of the dream . . . In other words, distortion was shown in this case to be deliberate and to be a means of *dissimulation*. My dream thoughts had contained a slander against R.; and, in order that I might not notice this, what appeared in the dream was the opposite, a feeling of affection for him.

(I, 140–141)

According to Freud, his Dream of the Uncle soothes his anxiety that, being Jewish, he may not be appointed to a well-deserved professorship. He traces the dream's infantile source to a prophecy of his future glory: instead of being turned down, he became the Minister of Education, the very official who hands out professorships. This dream wish presumably shows through the presence of two of Freud's professional friends, represented in the dream as similar to his uncle Josef, one of them being a simpleton, the other a criminal. Both of them are therefore suspect for the Minister, whereas Freud is quite unimpeachable. He can therefore expect to receive the professorship.

We need to reach beyond Freud's analysis. The death of his uncle Josef on 5 March 1897 occurred a month after Freud had received the news of his nomination (8 February 1897; see a letter to Fliess on that date). It seems to us that, given the dates, the uncle's death could just as easily have generated the dream as could the news of Freud's nomination. (Freud himself situates his dream in the spring of 1897, after both events.)[8] Freud says that he disguised Uncle Josef in the dream to distract himself from the anxiety of being rejected. In our opinion, the reverse is the case. The dream uses Freud's current apprehension about the professorship as a ploy, in an attempt to shield himself from the emotional impact of the family trauma that his uncle's death cannot have failed to revive in him.

We would like to point out Freud's aloofness in speaking of his uncle's "crime." Of Josef's misstep only the legal perspective seems to have survived, along with the characterization that he was a simpleton, as stated by his brother Jakob. We can only guess how intense the trauma must have been: Jakob's hair turned gray from grief. No sooner does Freud mention this fact than he tries to diminish its significance. He goes on to speak of the period of his uncle's imprisonment as a cheerful time, full of hope, the opposite of the dreary present. (At the time of his uncle's imprisonment, Freud was ten years old. He received the prophecy about his future glory when he was eleven or twelve.) Yet what is dreary for Freud in the present? Is it the rejection he anticipates because he is Jewish? While certainly justified under the Austro-Hungarian monarchy, can this worry compare with the public condemnation of Josef Freud? The past shaken by a family dishonor appears far more dreary than professional recognition in the present. Except if the shame persists, compromising ambition and lurking in the emotional background as a ghostly presence, ready to haunt the dreamer at any moment.

In his friend N., Freud wants to see a criminal, in R., a simpleton. In the dream these features supposedly cost his friends their professorships, but the unblemished Freud has reason to hope. This is the wish Freud would like to express to himself and his readers. What is the uneasiness hiding behind it? The Minister might turn down Freud because of his family, because of the crime committed by Josef Freud. To our ears this is the unspoken import of Freud's Dream of the Uncle.

A few more elements in the dream deserve closer attention, for example Freud's "excessive affection" for his friend R. "After the idea occurred to me that R. was my uncle, I had had a warm feeling of affection for him . . . I had naturally never had any feeling of affection for my Uncle Josef. I had been fond of my friend R . . . but if I had gone up to him and expressed . . . the degree of affection I had felt . . . in the dream, . . . he would have been astonished" (I, 140). Freud's unconscious fear that he may be denied the professorship because of his uncle provides new insight about the feeling of affection. We know from the news reports of the court proceedings that there were two defendants, Josef Freud and Osias Weich. The affection Sigmund Freud felt for his friend R. in the dream and that he found so puzzling (he returns to it four times in his associations) may have been an unwitting recollection. In the original German, affection is *Zärtlichkeit* and one of its synonyms is the word *Weich*heit, tenderness. Do Freud's dream thoughts hide Osias Weich's name? If so, why? The fact that Freud assigns the attributes of being a simpleton and a criminal to two separate people, his friends R. and N., may explain it. We capture here an indirect recollection of Jakob Freud's account to his nine-year-old son Sigmund in 1865: Your uncle is not a bad person, just a simpleton; Weich is the real criminal!

We no longer doubt that the unconscious core of Freud's

dream is a preoccupation with his uncle Josef. A simple but decisive hint confirms this interpretation. The first image of Freud's dream, *R. is my uncle,* sounds identical in German to *He is my uncle* (R = *er* = he). Freud's friends R. and N. appear in his dream to distract his attention from the sad memory of his stigmatized uncle. Another tangible token of the dream's latent significance—that Freud's desire to blot out his family's dishonor matches his extraordinary ambition of grandeur—shows in his use of words. He says of Uncle Josef that he had become a criminal because of his *eagerness for money* (138), and of himself he says that he is *eager for glory* (192). (Eager for money = *gewinn*sücht*ig*; eagerness for glory = *Grössensehn*sucht.)

Dream of Count Thun (Part II)

Date: August 1898

In the example which I shall next bring forward I have been able to catch the dream-work in the very act of intentionally fabricating an absurdity for which there was absolutely no occasion in the material. It is taken from the dream which arose from my meeting with Count Thun as I was starting for my holidays. *I was driving in a cab and ordered the driver to drive me to a station. "Of course, I can't drive with you along the railway line itself," I said, after he had raised some objection, as though I had overtired him. It was as if I had already driven with him for some of the distance one normally travels by train.* The analysis produced the following explanations of this confused and senseless story. The day before, I had hired a cab to take me to an out-of-the-way street in Dornbach. The driver, however, had not known where the street was and, as these excellent people are apt to do, had driven on and on until at last I had noticed what was happening and had told him the right way . . . We are now to discover the significance of absurdity in dreams and the motives which lead to its being admitted or even created. The solution to the mystery in the present dream was as follows. It was necessary for me that there should be something absurd and unintelligible in this dream in connection with the word *fahren* [to drive (in a cab); to travel (for example, in a train)] because the dream-thoughts included a particular judgment which called for representation. One evening, while I was at the house of the hospitable and witty lady who appeared as the "housekeeper" in one of the other scenes in the same dream, I had heard two riddles which I had been unable to solve. Since they were familiar to the rest of the company, I cut a rather ludicrous figure in my vain attempts to find the answers. They depended upon puns on the words *Nachkommen* [come after; descendants] and *Vorfahren* [to drive up; ancestors] and, I believe, ran as follows:

> With the master's request
> The driver complies
> By all men possessed
> In the graveyard it lies.

(Answer: drive up; ancestors = *Vorfahren*)

It was particularly confusing that the first half of the second riddle was identical with that of the first:

> With the master's request
> The driver complies:
> Not by all men possessed
> In the cradle it lies.

(Answer: come after; descendants = *Nachkommen*)

When I saw Count Thun *drive up* so impressively and when I thereupon fell into the mood of Figaro, with his remarks on the goodness of great gentlemen in having taken the trouble to be born (to become *progeny*), these two riddles were adopted by the dream-work as intermediate thoughts . . . The dream-thought . . . ran as follows: "It is absurd to be proud of one's ancestry; it is better to be an ancestor oneself." This judgment, that something "is absurd," was what produced the absurdity in the dream . . . A dream is made absurd, then, if a judgment that something is "absurd" is among the elements included in the dream-thoughts—that is to say, if any one of the dreamer's unconscious trains of thought has criticism or ridicule as its motive.

(I, 431–434)

In the first part of his dream Freud rejoices in a sense of revolutionary triumph as he indulges his sudden urge to hum Figaro's air from Mozart's opera, mocking the nobility of birth. By the end of his associations Freud reaches the point of wanting to rid himself of his ancestors. However, he forgets to explain why. This question will guide our interpretation.

Two of Freud's dreams concerning his dead father (who died in 1896) frame his Dream of Count Thun in *The Interpretation of Dreams*. In the dream called Father on His Deathbed, the dreamer says, *"I remembered how like Garibaldi he had looked on his death-bed"* (I, 428). Garibaldi's first name was Giuseppe = Joseph. Moreover, at the very beginning of his Dream of Count Thun (I, 211), Freud mentions the fiftieth jubilee of Emperor Franz-Josef of Austria. Thus Freud directly and indirectly identifies the apparently nameless ancestors, putting particular emphasis on the name *Joseph*. This leads us to believe that with his Dream of Count Thun Freud provides a sequel to his Dream of the Uncle. While the Dream of the Uncle shows us Freud being anxious about his future professorship—will the authorities use Uncle Josef's criminal record to block the nephew?—the glee running through the Dream of Count Thun brushes aside every bit of worry. The best way to attain glory on your own merit is to get rid of your ancestors!

The critical judgment about his forebears—"It is absurd to be proud about one's ancestry; it is better to be an ancestor oneself"

(I, 434)—seems to Freud a sufficient explanation of the dream's absurd form. Still, the documents about his uncle's counterfeiting affair take us further afield. The apparently senseless elements of the dream's second half—a lost cabdriver and riddles involving compounds of the German word *fahren:* to travel or take a cab—allow us to see an ancestor's unfortunate story. "The cabdriver did not know the way," in short, he lost his way. To lose one's way is translated by *verfahren* in German. This word means *going astray,* both literally and figuratively. It also resonates in German with one of the solutions to the riddle Freud could not answer, namely *forebears: Vorfahren.* If we link the two words, we read: a forebear has gone to the bad. The dreamer's claim that ancestors are a useless lot is now clear in relation to Freud's own family situation: he wants to get free from Josef, an ancestor who has gone astray. Freud wants to throw off the dishonor he has inherited.

The second half of his dream seems confused and absurd to Freud. According to him, the dream-work intentionally fabricated an absurd *form* so as to suggest the latent *content* of his judgment regarding ancestors. Yet no real absurdity exists once we translate the image of the lost cabdriver with the expression "he has gone astray" *(verfahren)* and if in turn we apply this expression to a shameful "ancestor" *(Vorfahren)* of Freud's, Uncle Josef. (By the way, Freud indirectly recalls his uncle's trial with the ambiguous term "judgment.") The only absurdity here would be the fact of being unjustly held accountable for the misdeeds of one's ancestors. In his Dream of Count Thun Freud rebels against the socially and professionally embarrassing or harmful effects of his uncle's crime.

The Dream of Non Vixit

Another dream, *Non vixit,* renews the attempt to shake off Uncle Josef's crime. Freud communicates his latent dream thoughts: he has the power to annihilate ghosts from the past with a look, or he can simply wish them away. We will peek behind Freud's sense of satisfaction—he survives all his dead or estranged friends, and he is finally unrivaled in possession of the field—at the series of public places and figures in the dream that bear the name Joseph. The Dream of *Non vixit,* in which so many different people named Joseph appear, reveals an unacknowledged and painful emotional reality for Freud. No matter how fervently he would wish it, he cannot dispel the eternal and ghostly return of an unspoken family trauma.

It is useful to summarize this exceptionally long dream before reading some excerpts. Freud worries about his friend Fliess, who will soon be undergoing surgery. At the same time, Freud participates in the unveiling of a memorial bust of one of his deceased friends, Fleischl. In a different image, the dreamer sees the ghost of another deceased friend (Paneth) with Fliess in a café and then makes the ghost disappear. His thoughts about his deceased friends remind Freud of a whole series of dead figures whom he has survived. He also tells of his feelings toward them: nobody is irreplaceable. In addition, Freud mentions all sorts of people, streets, and monuments named Joseph, a name he considers crucial in his life. Yet behind the series of friends and public places bearing the name Joseph, he sees John, his nephew living in England, with whom, as a child, he had a stormy friendship, born simultaneously of hate and love.

Excerpts from Freud's Dream of *Non vixit* and his associations:

Date: October 1898

I had a very clear dream. *I had gone to Brücke's laboratory at night, and, in response to a gentle knock on the door, I opened it to* (the late) *Professor Fleischl* . . . This was followed by a second dream. *My friend Fl.* [Fliess] *had come to Vienna unobtrusively in July. I met him in the street in conversation with my* (deceased) *friend P.,* . . . *Fl spoke about his sister and* *said that in three-quarters of an hour she was dead . . . As P. failed to understand him, Fl. turned to me and asked how much I had told P. about his affairs. Whereupon, overcome by strange emotions, I tried to explain to Fl. that P. (could not understand anything at all, of course, because he) was not alive. But what I actually said—and I myself noticed the mistake—was, "*NON VIXIT*." *I then gave P. a piercing look. Under my gaze he . . . melted away. I was highly delighted at this and I now realized that Ernst Fleischl, too, had been no more than an apparition, a "revenant"* [ghost—literally, one who returns]; *and it seemed to me quite possible that people of that kind only existed as long as one liked and could be got rid of if someone else wished it.*

This fine specimen includes many of the characteristics of dreams—the fact that I exercised my critical faculties during the dream and myself noticed my mistake when I said *"Non vixit"* instead of *"Non vivit"* [that is, "he did not live" instead of "he is not alive"], my unconcerned dealings with people who were dead and were recognized as being dead in the dream itself, the absurdity of my final inference and the great satisfaction it gave me . . . The central feature of the dream was a scene in which I annihilated P. with a look . . . This scene was unmistakably copied from one which I had actually experienced. At the time I have in mind I had been a demonstrator at the Physiological Institute and was due to start work early in the morning. It came to Brücke's ears that I sometimes reached the students' laboratory late . . . What overwhelmed me were the terrible blue eyes with which he looked at me and by which I was reduced to nothing—just as P. was in the dream, where, to my relief, the roles were reversed . . .

It was a long time, however, before I succeeded in tracing the origin of *"Non vixit"* with which I passed judgement in the dream. But at last it occurred to me that these two words possessed their high degree of clarity in the dream, not as words heard or spoken, but as words *seen*. I then knew at once where they came from. On the pedestal of the Kaiser Josef Memorial in the Hofburg [Imperial Palace] in Vienna the following impressive words are inscribed: "Saluti patriae vixit non diu sed totus [For his country's well-being he lived not long but wholly]." I extracted from this inscription just enough to fit in with a hostile train of ideas among the dream-thoughts, just enough to imply that "this fellow has no say in the matter—he isn't even alive." And this reminded me that I had the dream only a few days after the unveiling of the memorial to Fleischl in the cloisters of the University. At that time I had seen the Brücke memorial once again and must have reflected (unconsciously) with regret on the fact that the premature death of my brilliant friend P., whose whole life had been devoted to science, had robbed him of a well-merited claim to a memorial in these same precincts. Accordingly, I gave him this memorial in my dream; and, incidentally, as I remembered, his first name was Josef. [Footnote inserted here by Freud: I may add as an example of over-determination that my excuse for arriving too late at the laboratory lay in the fact that after working far into the night I had in the morning to cover the long distance between the *Kaiser Josef* Strasse and the Währinger Strasse.] (I, 421–423)

I once acted in the scene between Brutus and Caesar from Schiller before an audience of children. I was fourteen years old at the time and was acting with a nephew who was a year my senior. He had come to us on a visit from England; and he, too, was a *revenant* [a ghost], for it was the playmate of my earliest years who had returned in him. Until the end of my third year we had been inseparable. We had loved each other and fought with each other . . . Since that time my nephew John has had many reincarnations which revived now one side and now another of his personality, unalterably fixed as it was in my unconscious memory. There must have been times when he treated me very badly and I must have shown courage in the face of my tyrant; for in my later years I have often been told of a short speech made by me in my own defence when my father, who was at the same time John's grandfather, had said to me accusingly: "Why are you hitting John?" My reply—I was not yet two years old at the time—was "I hit him 'cos he hit me." It must have been this scene from my childhood which diverted *"Non vivit"* into *"Non vixit,"* for in the language of later childhood the word for to hit is *"wichsen"* [pronounced like the English "vixen"]. The dream-work is not ashamed to make use of links such as this one. There was little basis in reality for my hostility to my friend P., who was very greatly my superior and for that reason was well fitted to appear as a new edition of my early playmate. This hostility must therefore certainly have gone back to my complicated childhood relations to John. (I, 424–425)

We can gain a little insight into . . . a dream of which the words *"Non vixit"* formed the centre-point. In that dream manifestations of affect of various qualities were brought together at two points in its manifest content. Hostile and distressing feelings . . . were piled up at the point at which I annihilated my opponent and friend with two words. And again, at the end of the dream, I was highly delighted, and I went on to approve the possibility, which in waking life I knew was absurd, of there being *revenants* who could be eliminated by a mere wish.

I have not yet related the exciting cause of the dream. It was of great importance and led deep into an understanding of the dream. I had heard from my friend in Berlin, whom I have referred to as "Fl" [Fliess], that he was about to undergo an operation . . . The first reports . . . were not reassuring . . . I should have much preferred to go to him myself, but just at the time I was the victim of a painful complaint which made movement of any kind a torture to me. The dream-thoughts now informed me that I feared for my friend's life. His only sister . . . died in early youth after a brief illness . . .

Along with the unfavourable reports during the first few days after the operation, I was given a warning not to discuss the matter with anyone . . . I was very disagreeably affected by the veiled reproach because it was—not wholly without justification . . . I caused trouble between two friends . . . by quite unnecessarily telling one of them . . . what the other had said about him. At that time, too, reproaches had been levelled at me, and they were still in my memory. One of the two friends concerned was Professor Fleischl; I may describe the second by his first name of "Josef" [Breuer]— which was also that of P., my friend and opponent in the dream. (I, 480–482)

My present-day anger, which was only slight, over the warning I had been given not to give anything away [about Fliess's illness] received reinforcements from sources in the depth of my mind . . . The source . . . flowed from my childhood . . . [It] went back to my relations in childhood with a nephew . . . we were inseparable friends, and . . . we sometimes fought with each other . . . All my friends have in a certain sense been re-incarnations of this first figure . . .: they have been *revenants* . . . It has not infrequently happened that the ideal situation of childhood has been so completely reproduced that friend and enemy have come together in a single individual . . .

From this point the dream-thoughts proceeded along some such lines as these: "It serves you right if you had to make way for me. Why did you try to push *me* out of the way? I don't need you, I can easily find someone else to play with," and so on. These thoughts now entered upon the paths which led to their representation in the dream. There had been a time when I had had to reproach my friend Josef [P.] for an attitude of this same kind . . . But, as was to be expected, the dream punished my friend, and not me, for this callous wish. [Footnote inserted here by Freud: It will be noticed that the name Josef plays a great part in my dreams (cf. the dream about my uncle). My own ego finds it very easy to hide itself behind people of that name, since Joseph was the name of a man famous in the Bible as an interpreter of dreams.]

"As he was ambitious, I slew him" . . . Thus a part of the satisfaction I felt in the dream was to be interpreted: "A just punishment! It serves you right!" . . .

Thus it seemed to me quite natural that the *revenants* should only exist for just so long as one likes and should be removable at a wish. We have seen what my friend Josef was punished for. But the *revenants* were a series of reincarnations of the friend of my childhood. It was therefore also a source of satisfaction to me that I had always been able to find successive substitutes for that figure; and I felt . . .: no one was irreplaceable . . .

In addition to this, however, the dream contained a clear allusion to another train of thought which could legitimately lead to satisfaction. A short time before, after long expectation, a daughter had been born to my friend [Fliess] . . . My friend's baby daughter had the same name as the little girl I used to play with as a child, who was of my age and the sister of my earliest friend and opponent . . . From here my thoughts went on to the subject of the names of my own children. I had insisted on their names being chosen, not according to the fashion of the moment but in memory of people I have been fond of. Their names made the children into *revenants*. And, after all, I reflected, was not having children our only path to immortality? (I, 480–487)

How does Freud interpret his dream? I had a very dear childhood friend, my nephew John. We both loved each other and fought with each other. Hence my feelings of ambivalence and rivalry toward all my other friends and colleagues, actually all of them reincarnations of John. So they are ghosts in a sense. Their death even reassures me; I've survived them all. If they were ever to return, for example in my dreams, I would have the power to annihilate them at my discretion. This idea makes me happy. In any case, they deserve their punishment. When they were alive, they tried to bully me, to kick me out of my rightful place. Ultimately, I will survive even my own death thanks to the immortality my descendants will supply.

Let us go further than Freud with the question: Is someone or something dead, a ghost, living on in Freud—but without his knowledge? Freud isolates John, his nephew, as the childhood figure hiding behind all his subsequent friends. Yet, besides this meaning, or perhaps in contradiction with it, Freud also brings up many a time the name Joseph. Taking into account the new biographical material relating to Josef Freud—and especially the Uncle Dream, to which Freud makes special reference in his associations—Uncle Josef might appear more significant in the dream's creation than nephew John. In attributing a decisive influence to his nephew, is Freud seeking to cast off his uncle's hold over him? Indeed, the very relationship of uncle to nephew between Sigmund and John Freud provides us with an additional interpretive clue.[9] John's presence hints at the problem bound up with an uncle, constantly recalled by the many occurrences of the name Joseph. Of course, Freud's experiences (at age two or three) with his nephew John do precede by several years Uncle Josef's arrest and imprisonment, but this does not give John any priority. Freud's reversal of the emotional significance of these two facts— the warlike childhood friendship and the painful family dishonor—is no doubt the work of unconscious censorship.

The Dream of *Non vixit* heightens the subject of the Dream of Count Thun. The wish to throw off one's ancestors expands with the desire to annihilate ghosts. Let us recall a few dates. Uncle Josef died in March 1897; the dreams of Count Thun and *Non vixit* are respectively from August and October of the following year. The year and a half that elapsed after Uncle Josef's death probably proved too little time for Freud to mourn the memory of someone whose actions had once upon a time led to a painful family atmosphere of stifled shame.

"It will be noticed that the name Josef plays a great part in my dreams (cf. the dream about my uncle). My own ego finds it very easy to hide itself behind people of that name, since Joseph was the name of a man famous in the Bible as an interpreter of dreams." The name Josef reappears in six different contexts in Freud's dream: Josef Paneth, Freud's dead friend; Emperor Franz-Josef's monument; Josef Breuer; Joseph, the biblical interpreter of dreams; Uncle Josef; the Kaiser-Josef Strasse. This abundance of the name Joseph works as a sign of insistence. Some Joseph is being summoned by all manner of means. Which Joseph is it? The biblical interpreter of dreams, with whom Freud so willingly identifies? We do not think so. The biblical Joseph stands in rather more for the uncle. Both went to prison, but one was guilty, the other innocent. The one fell, the other rose to glory. The idealized image of a biblical Joseph, covered with honors, is, alas, no more than make-believe. Uncle Josef's shameful crime is the all too distressing reality. It is his misstep that refuses to dissipate with a simple look, or melt away at a wish.

Freud's own mistake in substituting the past tense *non vixit* (he *did not* live) for the present (he *is not* living) bears this out. According to Freud's interpretation, the sound pattern of the Latin word *vixit* derives from the German word for beating: *wichsen,* a recollection of his stormy relationship with his nephew John. However, Freud ties his direct and visual recollection to someone named Josef:

> It occurred to me that these two words [*non vixit*] possessed their high degree of clarity in the dream not as words heard or spoken, but as words seen . . . On the pedestal of the Kaiser Josef Memorial in the Hofburg [Imperial Palace] in Vienna the following impressive words are inscribed: Saluti patriae vixit non diu [For the well-being of his country he *lived not* long] . . . I extracted from this inscription just enough to fit in with the hostile train of ideas among the dream-thoughts, just enough to imply that "this fellow [Josef Paneth] has nothing to say in the matter—he isn't even alive."

Sure enough, Freud's dead friend Josef Paneth will not disturb him any more; Freud has no trouble making his ghost disappear. Will it be as easy for him to repel the specter of Uncle Josef? Most likely not. Of the uncle the dreamer would prefer to say: he did not live—*non vixit.* This error bares Freud's deepest and most censored wish. Would that Uncle Josef had never existed! That way, he wouldn't have been able to bring shame and misfortune on the family. If Freud has little reason to bother with his friend Paneth—whoever is dead should keep his mouth shut!—he lacks that kind of freedom when it comes to his uncle. Making an obvious mistake about him—he did not live—Freud says that his uncle refuses to keep silent in him. Josef survives as a ghost, he lives on beyond the grave as a haunting presence for his nephew. So, the Dream of *Non vixit* restates in ever stronger terms Freud's desire to rid himself of his ancestors (see his Dream of Count

Thun). If his relatives had never existed, there would be no need for Freud to tolerate their disturbing visitations from the grave.

The Dream of *Non vixit* raises a paradoxical memorial to Josef Freud. Instead of celebrating him: He lived, he accomplished so much . . ., the dream inscribes on the pedestal, *He lived—No!* This indicates to what extent Freud was unable to bury his uncle. Josef stays with him as an affliction, a painful complaint, a torture, a *furuncle*. These are the very words of Freud's dream: "I was the victim of a painful complaint which made movement of any kind a torture to me" (I, 480–481). Another dream, Riding on a Horse, will tie the pain to the uncle.

Dream of Riding on a Horse

Both Riding on a Horse and *Non Vixit* mention Freud's boils, and in very similar terms: "For some days before I had been suffering from boils [*Furunkel*] which made every movement a torture" (I, 230); "I was the victim of a painful complaint which made movement of any kind a torture to me" (I, 480–481).[10]

Excerpts from Freud's Dream of Riding on a Horse and his interpretation:

Date: October 1898

I was riding on a grey horse, timidly and awkwardly to begin with . . . I met one of my colleagues, P., who was sitting high on a horse . . . and who drew my attention to something (probably to my bad seat). I now began to find myself sitting more and more firmly . . . and noticed that I was feeling quite at home up there. My saddle was a kind of bolster . . . Then I actually did dismount . . . My hotel was in the same street; I might have let the horse go to it on its own, but I preferred to lead it there. It was as though I should have felt ashamed to arrive at it on horseback. A hotel "boots" was standing in front of the hotel; he showed me a note of mine that had been found . . . In the note was written, doubly underlined: "No food," and then another remark (indistinct) *such as "No work" . . .*

For some days before I had been suffering from boils which made every movement a torture; and finally a boil the size of an apple had risen at the base of my scrotum, which caused me the most unbearable pain with every step I took . . . I was not properly capable of discharging my medical duties. There was, however, one activity for which, in view of the nature and situation of my complaint, I should certainly have been less fitted than for any other, and that was—riding. And this was precisely the activity in which the dream landed me: it was the most energetic denial of my illness [suffering] that could possibly be imagined . . . But in this dream I was riding as though I had no boil on my perineum—or rather *because I wanted not to have one.* My saddle, to judge from the description, was the poultice which had made it possible for me to fall asleep. Under its assuaging influence I had probably been unaware of my pain during the first hours of sleep. The painful feelings then announced themselves and sought to wake me; whereupon the dream came and said soothingly: "No! Go on sleeping! There's no need to wake up. You haven't got a boil; for you're riding a horse, and it's quite certain that you couldn't ride if you had a boil in that particular place." And the dream was successful. The pain was silenced, and I went on sleeping . . .

My friend P. liked to ride *the high horse* with me ever since he had taken over one of my women patients . . . *"I felt quite at home up there"* referred to the position I had occupied in this patient's house before I was replaced by P. Not long before, one of my few patrons among the leading physicians in this city had remarked to me in connection with this same house: "You struck me as being firmly in the saddle there."

It was a remarkable *feat*, too, to be able to carry on my psychotherapeutic work for eight or ten hours a day while I was having so much pain. But I knew that I could not go on long with my peculiarly difficult work unless I was in completely sound physical health; and my dream was full of gloomy allusions to the situation in which I should then find myself. (The *note . . . no work, no food*.) In the course of further interpretation I saw that the dream-work had succeeded in finding a path from the wishful situation of riding to some scenes of quarreling from my very early childhood which must have occurred between me and a nephew of mine, a year my senior, who was at present living in England. Furthermore, the dream had derived some of its elements from my travels in Italy; the street in the dream was composed of impressions of Verona and Siena. A still deeper interpretation led to sexual dream-thoughts, and I recalled the meaning which references to Italy seem to have had in the dreams of a woman patient who had never visited that lovely country: *"gen Italien"* [to Italy]—*"Genitalien"* [genitals]; and this was connected, too, with the . . . situation of my boil. (I, 229–232)

In his interpretation, Freud points to the painful abscess that his dream was supposed to silence so that he could go on sleeping. He also proposes a sexual interpretation, based on the location of his boil under the scrotum.

The terms of the dream and the associations allow us to conjecture an additional layer of signification. Freud uses the word *Furunkel* = furuncle seven times and not *Abzess* = abscess or another German synonym of boil, such as *Blutgeschwür*. Undoubtedly real, the physical ailment also reactivates psychic events for Freud. In his painful fur*uncle*, we hear a painful complaint about Uncle Josef. Freud would like to think that his dream can soothe his current distress, his painful boil, but the words he uses in his dream text and associations outline, in anagrammatic form, his uncle's criminal past. Thus the bandage placed on the site of his bodily pain will not suffice to silence the underlying emotional affliction.

> I was not properly capable of discharging my medical duties. There was, however, one activity for which, in view of the nature and situation of my complaint, I should certainly have been less fitted than for any other, and that was riding . . . But in this dream I was riding as though I had no furuncle on my perineum—rather because *I wanted not to have one.* My saddle, to judge from its description, was the poultice which had made it possible for me to fall asleep.

In this account, verbal fragments hint at Uncle Josef's criminal activities: he passes or *spreads* counterfeit money. *Horse, poultice, bandage,* and *riding* together delineate the word *spreads* in German. (*Pferd:* horse, *Brei*umschlag: poultice, *reitet:* rides = *fer-brei-reitet* = *verbreitet:* he spreads; in German the sounds *f* and *v* are interchangeable.) Other elements in the dream suggest Freud's emotional state. "*Then I actually did dismount . . . My hotel was in the same street; I might have let the horse go to it on its own, but I preferred to lead it there. It was as though I should have felt ashamed to arrive at it on horseback.*" Once again Freud provides a verbal fragment of his uncle's activities (rider: *Reiter:* Verbreiter: peddler), and tells of his own shame. We can also hear a hidden reference to his uncle's imprisonment in the painful furuncle's twofold description: "for some days before I had been suffering from furuncles which made every movement a torture" and "I was the victim of a painful complaint which made movement of any kind a torture to me." As before, perceive *uncle* on the one hand and *he is in prison* on the other. Fur*uncle* suggests the painful uncle and *victim* of a painful complaint hints at his imprisonment. (A fragment of the German original of victim: *behaftet* means *arrest* = *Haft,* and recalls *Haft*anstalt: prison.)

"The dream . . . was the most energetic denial of my suffering that could possibly be imagined." This is Freud's ardent wish. It is also his response to the unconscious source of his anguish: if known, his uncle's crime and imprisonment could land him in trouble with his patients, making him lose his livelihood. Freud says that people thought he had been firmly in the saddle, but he was actually doing poorly. He goes on to imagine the dire consequences: no work, no food. Suffering from a painful furuncle, really from an uncle convicted once upon a time as a criminal, does Freud fear the worst for his career and reputation? This latent anxiety uses the bodily pain as a means for expressing the psychological burden. Freud's apprehension here connects directly with his Dream of the Uncle. The specter of Josef's crime threatens to deprive Sigmund not only of his well-deserved professorship but also of all other forms of professional success. What will come of all that? Shame, misery, and destitution? Freud fears his uncle's prison, he agonizes over the unconscious thought of being forever confined to Josef's ill-fated past.

Dream of the Open-air Closet

The Dream of the Open-Air Closet appears far more optimistic; it discards as rubbish all anxiety about the uncle. Excerpts from Freud's dream and associations:

Date: August 1898
A hill on which there was something like an open-air closet: a very long seat with a large hole at the end of it. Its back edge was thickly covered with small heaps of faeces of all sizes and degrees of freshness. There were bushes behind the seat. I mictu-

rated on the seat; a long stream of urine washed everything clean; the lumps of faeces came away easily and fell into the opening. It was as though at the end there was still some left.

Why did I feel no disgust during this dream?

Because, as the analysis showed, the most agreeable and satisfying thoughts contributed to bringing the dream about. What at once occurred to me in the analysis were the Augean stables which were cleansed by Hercules. This Hercules was I . . . The seat (except, of course, for the hole) was an exact copy of a piece of furniture which had been given to me as a present by a grateful woman patient. It thus reminded me of how much my patients honoured me . . . The stream of urine which washed everything clean was an unmistakable sign of greatness. It was in that way that Gulliver extinguished the great fire in Lilliput . . . But Gargantua, too, Rabelais' superman, revenged himself in the same way on the Parisians by sitting astride on Notre Dame and turning his stream of urine upon the city . . . And strangely enough, here was another piece of evidence that I was a superman. The platform of Notre Dame was my favourite resort in Paris . . . The fact that all the faeces disappeared so quickly under the stream recalled the motto: "Afflavit et dissipati sunt" [He blew and they were scattered], which I intended one day to put at the head of a chapter upon the therapy of hysteria.

And now for the true exciting cause of the dream. It had been a hot summer afternoon; and during the evening I had delivered my lecture on the connection between hysteria and the perversions, and everything I had had to say displeased me intensely and seemed to me completely devoid of any value . . . I longed to be away from all this grubbing about in human dirt . . . In this mood I went from the lecture room to a café . . . One of my audience, however, went with me . . . He began to flatter me: telling me how much he had learnt from me, how he looked at everything now with fresh eyes, how I had cleansed the *Augean stables* of errors and prejudices in my theory of the neuroses. He told me, in short, that I was a very great man. My mood fitted ill with this paean of praise; . . . before going to sleep I turned over the pages of Rabelais and read one of Conrad Ferdinand Meyer's short stories, *"Die Leiden eines Knaben"* [A Boy's Sorrows].

Such was the material out of which the dream emerged. Meyer's short story brought up in addition a recollection of scenes from my childhood. (Cf. the last episode in the dream about Count Thun.) The day-time mood of revulsion and disgust persisted into the dream in so far as it was able to provide almost the entire material of its manifest content. But during the night a contrary mood of powerful and even exaggerated self-assertiveness arose and displaced the former one. The content of the dream had to find a form which would enable it to express both the delusions of inferiority and the megalomania in the same material.   (I, 468–470)

Freud's interpretation is clear. A feeling of inferiority, fed by both recent and infantile sources, gives way to self-satisfaction. Freud's contributions to the theory of the neuroses will make him a great man, no, a superman, like Gulliver, Gargantua, or Hercules. Freud indicates a dynamic relationship between his contrary feelings of worthlessness and conceit: his delusion of grandeur washes everything clean. However, he does not say why, in order to assert his value fully, it is necessary to clear away excrement and dirt. This question directs our analysis.

At the close of his associations, Freud simply mentions a short story by Conrad Ferdinand Meyer, a Swiss author, without hinting at its content. (An extended summary of it can be found in

Grinstein's *On Sigmund Freud's Dreams,* pp. 437–440.) On reading "A Boy's Sorrows" we feel encouraged to search for an
unconscious motivation behind Freud's desire for grandeur amid
the surrounding filth. Meyer's tale relates the demise of young
Julien Boufflers, a pupil in a Jesuit school who is hounded to
death by his teachers when his father uncovers the Jesuits' fraudulent machinations in a financial transaction and later refuses to
hand over the incriminating documents. Meyer's story clarifies
Freud's underlying dream wish. No longer a boy like the unfortunate Julien Boufflers, Freud will not accept being an impotent
victim of the fraudulent manipulations going on around him.
Sigmund will know how to wash away the dirt that besmirched
the name Freud. He will be like a giant, a superman, even a god,
if need be, to restore his family's stained honor.

Verbal elements in the dream deepen our interpretation. To
clean away the litter, Freud urinates on a seat or bench, in German
a *Bank,* a homonym of the German and English bank or financial
institution. The *back edge* of the bench [*die hintere Kante der
Bank*] is covered with heaps of excrement. This formulation leads
us in two directions. First, there is dirt behind [*hinter*] the bench
or the *bank*. Second, the German original of *edge: Kante* recalls
the colloquial German expression for *saving or putting money
aside: Geld auf die höhe Kante legen.* The dirt that requires Freud's
nearly superhuman effort at removal relates to money and a bank.
Is this a hidden reference to Uncle Josef? Let us recall the letters
found on Josef in which his nephews asked him "to find a bank
for the merchandise where the turn-over would be larger, faster,
and more profitable."

In his associations Freud links his Dream of the Open-Air
Closet to his dream of Count Thun. The same Latin motto does
indeed appear in both. The motto, *Afflavit et dissipati sunt:* He
blew and they were scattered, is engraved on a medal commemo-
rating the victory of the English navy over the Spanish Armada

in 1588. In the context of the dreams we have just analyzed, with this motto Freud triumphantly dismisses his Uncle Josef's criminal past. In fact, when we combine the gist of a whole series of interconnected dreams (Dream of the Uncle, *Non vixit*, Count Thun, Riding on a Horse, Open-Air Closet), we arrive at the following unconscious speech: I, Sigmund Freud, will not be the helpless victim of my ancestors' misdeeds. It is true that I hurt because of my uncle's dirty money deals and continue to fear for my professional advancement. Still, if he tried to disturb me, I am quite sure that I could annihilate him. After all, he is dead, isn't he? I can surely dissipate this ghost of an affair constantly nagging me—but, of course, only if I say and believe that my uncle never existed at all. Everything opens up then; my professional and personal greatness manages to wash everything absolutely clean. Never again will I have to suffer like the powerless child that I was when my uncle Josef was caught red-handed and convicted, when he unsettled the entire family.

Dream of the Botanical Monograph

The Dream of the Botanical Monograph will reinforce the same assertion of free will, while latently revealing why this "freedom" to succeed is in fact a vital and inescapable obligation for Freud. This dream gives rise to an exceptionally intense analysis in *The Interpretation of Dreams*. Freud returns to it no fewer than seven times, enriching his dream with theoretical reflections on the role of displacement and condensation, on the suppression of affect as well as on the importance of significant infantile elements in dream interpretation. We will consider Freud's theoretical additions as part and parcel of his dream associations. In the same way, the many recurrences of this dream encourage us to use its immediate surroundings as a further source of associations.

Freud interprets his dream as follows. He saw a monograph on the genus cyclamen in a shop window. He regrets not having pursued his research into the properties of another plant, coca (the source of cocaine), the subject of one of his earliest scientific monographs. Behind the insignificant facade of the shop window lurks Freud's pride at having facilitated an important discovery of cocaine's anesthetic properties. It is hurt pride, however, because Freud's contribution seems not to have been fully acknowledged. The infantile source of his dream goes back to an early episode or screen memory: Freud pulls apart the pages of a book like the leaves of an artichoke. In the end, he is surprised at the dream's emotional indifference when in fact its subject—his freedom to act, to live as he likes and sees fit—would require a greater degree of intensity. (Freud says, "For reasons with which we are not concerned, I shall not pursue the interpretation of this dream any further"—I, 173. We find it unfruitful to speculate on the direction in which Freud might have taken the interpretation.)

Excerpts from Freud's Dream of the Botanical Monograph and his interpretation:

Date: 10 March 1898

I had written a monograph on a certain plant. The book lay before me and I was at the moment turning over a folded coloured plate. Bound up in each copy there was a dried specimen of the plant, as though it had been taken from a herbarium.

ANALYSIS

That morning I had seen a new book in the window of a book-shop, bearing the title *Genus cyclamen*—evidently a *monograph* on that plant.

Cyclamen, I reflected, were my wife's *favourite flowers* and I reproached myself for so rarely remembering to *bring* her *flowers*, which was what she liked.—The subject of *bringing flowers* recalled an anecdote which I had used as evidence in favour of my theory that forgetting is very often determined by an unconscious purpose and that it always enables one to deduce the secret intentions of the person who forgets. A young woman was accustomed to receiving a bouquet of flowers from her husband on her birthday. One year this token of his affection failed to appear, and she burst into tears . . . He clasped his hands to his head and exclaimed: . . . I'll go out at once and fetch your *flowers* . . . This lady, Frau L., had met my wife two days before I had had the dream . . .

I now made a fresh start. Once, I recalled, I really *had* written something in the nature of a *monograph on a plant,* namely a dissertation on the *coca plant,* which had drawn Karl Koller's attention to the anaesthetic properties of cocaine. I had myself indicated this application of the alkaloid in my published paper, but I had not been thorough enough to pursue the matter further . . . Shortly after Koller's discovery my father had in fact been attacked by glaucoma; my friend Dr. Königstein, the ophthalmic surgeon, had operated on him; while Dr. Koller had been in charge of the cocaine anaesthesia and had commented on the fact that this case had brought together all of the three men who had had a share in the introduction of cocaine.

My thoughts then went on to the occasion when I had last been reminded of this business of the cocaine. It had been a few days earlier, when I had been looking at a copy of a *Festschrift* in which grateful pupils had celebrated the jubilee of their teacher and laboratory director. Among the laboratory's claims to distinction which were enumerated in this book I had seen a mention of the fact that Koller had made his discovery there of the anaesthetic properties of cocaine. I then suddenly perceived that my dream was connected with an event of the previous evening. I had walked home precisely with Dr. Königstein . . . While I was talking to him in the entrance hall, Professor *Gärtner* [Gardener] and his wife had joined us; and I could not help congratulating them both on their *blooming* looks. But Professor Gärtner was one of the authors of the *Festschrift* I have just mentioned . . .

I will make an attempt at interpreting the other determinants of the content of the dream as well. There was *a dried specimen of the plant* included in the monograph, as though it had been a *herbarium*. This led me to a memory from my secondary school. Our headmaster once called together the boys from the higher forms and handed over the school's herbarium to them to be looked through and cleaned. Some small *worms*—bookworms—had found their way into it . . . In my preliminary examination in botany I was . . . given a Crucifer to identify—and failed to do so . . . I went on from the Cruciferae to the Compositae. It occurred to me that artichokes were Compositae, and indeed I might fairly have called them my *favourite flowers* . . .

The folded coloured plate. While I was a medical student I was the constant victim of an impulse only to learn things out of *monographs*. In spite of my limited means, I succeeded in getting hold of a number of volumes of the proceedings of medical societies and was enthralled by their *coloured plates* . . . There followed, I could not quite make out how, a recollection from very early youth. It had once amused my father to hand over a book with *coloured plates* (an account of a journey through Persia) for me and my eldest sister to destroy. Not easy to justify from the educational point of view! I had been five years old at the time and my sister not yet three; and the picture of the two of us blissfully pulling the book to pieces (leaf by leaf, like an *artichoke*) . . . Then, when I became a student, I had developed a passion for collecting and owning books . . . I had become a *book-worm* . . .

For reasons with which we are not concerned, I shall not pursue the interpretation of this any further, but will merely indicate the direction in which it lay . . . the dream . . . turns out to have been in the nature of a self-justification, a plea on behalf of my own rights . . . Even the apparently indifferent form in which the dream was couched turns out to have had significance. What it meant was: "After all, I'm the man who wrote the valuable and memorable paper (on cocaine)" . . . "I may allow myself to do this." (I, 169–173)

The dream-work has reduced to a level of indifference not only the content but often the emotional tone of my thoughts as well. It might be said that the dream-work brings about a *suppression of affects.* Let us, for instance, take the dream of the botanical monograph. The thoughts corresponding to it consisted of an agitated plea on behalf of my liberty to act as I chose to act and to govern my life as seemed right to me and me alone. The dream that arose from them has an indifferent ring about it . . . This reminds one of the peace that has descended upon a battlefield strewn with corpses; no trace is left of the struggle which raged over it.   (I, 467)

Note the discrepancy between the violent metaphors Freud associates with his dream and the rather more insignificant factors he sees at its root. We think that the dream's infantile motive as given, the book torn apart like an artichoke (an episode whose veracity as a recollection Freud goes on to dispute, see I, 173) is actually a displacement of a truly painful infantile experience, the counterfeiting affair; its unsettling emotional impact had been suppressed by Freud.

The context in which the dream appears in Freud's book sustains our hypothesis. His Dream of the Uncle frames the Botanical Monograph. No dream by Freud intervenes between the first account of his uncle dream (I, 136–145) and the Botanical Monograph (I, 169ff); similarly, the second account of the Botanical Monograph (I, 191) is followed directly by the second occurrence of the uncle dream (I, 192–193). Moreover, the last incarnation of the Botanical Monograph (I, 467) precedes the Dream of the Open-Air Closet (I, 468–470). These juxtapositions help us situate the source of the dream in the midst of Freud's family dishonor.

"Let us, for instance, take the dream of the botanical monograph. The thoughts corresponding to it consisted of a passionately agitated plea on behalf of my liberty to act and to govern my life as seemed right to me and to me alone. The dream that arose from them has an indifferent ring about it . . . This reminds me of the peace that has descended upon a battlefield strewn with corpses; no trace is left of the struggle which raged over it." We agree with Freud that his dream's indifference is the result of censorship. However, "the raging battlefield of corpses" (in Freud?) no doubt reaches deeper than the lack of recognition sustained by Freud in his work on the coca plant. We see here a similar problem to the one implied in Freud's Dream of the Open-Air Closet. There, Meyer's story "A Boy's Sorrows" hints at the Freud family's humiliation—to be washed clean by Sigmund's superhuman efforts. If he succeeds, he gains his freedom to act. For that he needs to cast off his ancestors or to silence their untoward and distressing ghostly returns (see the dreams of Count Thun and *Non vixit*). Can he do it? The Dream of the Botanical Monograph says he cannot.

Uncle Josef's unfortunate manipulations appear covertly among the multitude of flowers Freud mentions both in the Botanical Monograph and in his Dream of Count Thun. The

German names of two flowers, *violets* and *cyclamen,* occurring respectively in the two dreams, hide a secret meaning: *to counterfeit.* (This makes explicit our earlier contention that in his Dream of Count Thun Freud's intended revolution of dropping his burdensome relatives and of proclaiming himself his own ancestor is a response to his uncle's perennially troubling counterfeiting affair.) The path leading there in German is as follows. Violet = *Veilchen;* cyclamen = *Zyklamen,* but also the colloquial term *Alpenveilchen.* The Austrian-German pronunciation of *Veilchen* and *(Alpen)veilchen* sounds nearly identical to the verb *fälschen* = to counterfeit. In addition, the very word *flower*—constantly implied in Freud's many mentions of cyclamen, roses, tulips, carnations, colt's foot, the blooming looks of Mr. and Mrs. Gardener (Gärtner), his patient Flora, artichokes, his favorite flower—hides a German slang term, namely funny money = *Blüte* = flower.

Should we conclude, then, that Freud speaks the language of flowers (= *er spricht durch die Blume*) in the German sense of that expression, that is, that he speaks abstrusely, even for himself, when he talks about flowers in his dreams? Or better yet: Is Freud keeping from his notice a secret reference to *forged money* in the profusion of *flowers?* It is easier to understand now why Freud insists so vehemently on the importance of his work on the coca plant. *Do not look for any other flowers (Blüte = flower = Blüte = forged money)* in the Freud family apart from the coca plant. This one is glorious; it nearly made Sigmund Freud famous. Alas, the dream images do not lie. Their very indifference fails to erase their unsettling significance. Freud dreams of a book on *cyclamen,* a flower whose common German name contains the homonym of the word *to counterfeit.* To this dried flower, so unabashedly displayed for all to see in a shop window, corresponds perhaps another *pressed* flower, Uncle Josef's trial for selling counterfeit rubles, a trial so unhappily reported in the *press.*

Did the uncle's story of counterfeiting, this "dried flower," long since dead and apparently done with, undergo a "suppression of affect" in Freud? Cocaine's anesthetic properties, in part discovered by the dreamer himself and put to good use by his father's eye doctor, could perhaps work their magic on Sigmund Freud as well. This is, in our opinion, the dream's ultimate significance and Freud's secret hope. He would like to be anesthetized, so as not to hear himself ask who the dead are on the emotional "battlefield strewn with corpses," so as not to have to search for the hidden meaning of the battle raging within him.

The Nightmare of Self-dissection

Another dream, the Nightmare of Self-dissection, is much less capable of putting to rest the dreamer's anguish; it startles him with the dreadfulness of thinking. Excerpts from Freud's dream and interpretation:

Date: 1897–1899

*Old Brücke must have set me some ta*sk; STRANGELY ENOUGH, *it related to a dissection of the lower part of my own body, my pelvis and legs, which I saw before me as though in the dissecting-room, but without noticing their absence in myself and also without a trace of any gruesome feeling. Louise N. was standing beside me and doing the work with me. The pelvis had been eviscerated, and it was visible now in its superior, now in its inferior aspect, the two being mixed together. Thick flesh-coloured protuberances (which, in the dream itself, made me think of haemorrhoids) could be seen. Something which lay over it and was like crumpled silver-paper had also to be carefully fished out. I was then once more in possession of my legs and was making my way through the town. But (being tired) I took a cab. To my astonishment the cab drove in through the door of a house, which opened and allowed it to pass along a passage which turned a corner at its end and finally led into the open*

*air again. Finally I was making a journey through a chang-
ing landscape with an Alpine guide who was carrying my
belongings. Part of the way he carried me too, out of consideration for my tired legs. The ground was boggy; we went
round the edge; people were sitting on the ground like Indians
or gipsies—among them a girl. Before this I had been making
my own way forward over the slippery ground with a constant
feeling of surprise that I was able to do it so well after the
dissection. At last we reached a small wooden house at the end
of which was an open window. There the guide set me down
and laid two wooden boards, which were standing ready, upon
the window-sill, so as to bridge the chasm which had to be
crossed over from the window. At that point I really became
frightened about my legs, but instead of the expected crossing,
I saw two grown-up men lying on wooden benches that were
along the walls of the hut, and what seemed to be two children
sleeping beside them. It was as though what was going to make
the crossing possible was not the boards but the children. I
awoke in a mental fright.*

. . . The following was the occasion of the dream. Louise
N., the lady who was assisting me in my job in the dream,
had been calling on me. "Lend me something to read," she
had said. I offered her Rider Haggard's *She*. "A *strange*
book, but full of hidden meaning," I began to explain to
her; "the eternal feminine, the immortality of our emotions . . ." Here she interrupted me: "I know it already.
Have you nothing of your own?"—"No, my own immortal
works have not yet been written."—"Well, when are we to
expect these so-called ultimate explanations of yours . . . ?"
I reflected on the amount of self-discipline it was costing me
to offer the public even my book upon dreams—I should
have to give away so much of my own private character in
it.

Das Beste was du wissen kannst [The best of what you know],

Darfts den Buben doch nicht sagen [You cannot tell the boys].

The task which was imposed on me in the dream of carrying out a dissection of *my own body* was thus my *self-analysis* which was linked up with my giving an account of my dreams . . . The further thoughts which were started up by my conversation with Louise N. went too deep to become conscious. They were diverted in the direction of the material that had been stirred up by the mention of Rider Haggard's *She* . . . The boggy ground over which people had to be carried, and the chasm which they had to cross by means of boards brought along with them, were taken from *She;* the Red Indians, the girl and the wooden house were taken from *Heart of the World* [also by Rider Haggard]. Both novels . . . are concerned with perilous journeys; . . . *She* describes an adventurous road that had scarcely ever been trodden before, leading into an undiscovered region. The tired feeling in my legs, according to a note which I find I made upon the dream, had been a real sensation during the day-time. It probably went along with a tired mood and a doubting thought: "How much longer will my legs carry me?" The end of the adventure in *She* is that the guide, instead of finding immortality for herself and the others, perishes in the mysterious subterranean fire. A fear of that kind was unmistakably active in the dream-thoughts. The "wooden house" was also, no doubt, a coffin, that is to say, the grave. But the dream-work achieved a masterpiece in its representation of this most unwished-for of all thoughts by a wish-fulfillment. For I had already been in a grave once, but it was an excavated Etruscan grave near Orvieto . . . The dream seems to have been saying: "If you must rest in a grave, let it be the Etruscan one." And by making this replacement, it transformed the gloomiest of expectations into one that was highly desirable. Unluckily, as we are soon to hear [I, 460 ff], a dream can turn into its opposite the *idea* accompanying an affect but not always the affect itself. Accordingly, I woke up in a *"mental fright,"* even after the successful emergence of the idea that children may perhaps achieve what their father has failed to—a fresh allusion to the strange novel [*She*] in which a person's identity is retained through a series of generations for over two thousand years.   (I, 452–455)

Freud's interpretation is transparent. The dissection signifies the self-analysis he carries out by publishing his book on dreams. He has no gruesome feelings at all during the dissection because of his desire to keep under control the unpleasant aspects of his self-analysis. Moreover, he turns the gloomy prospect of his own death into its contrary with the thought that children might achieve what their father could not. Freud explains his fright upon awakening with the dream's inability to transform the affect of anticipated death into something more agreeable.

The dream elements lead us further on. It is certainly no mere coincidence that Freud's self-analysis should appear in a nightmare. What terror might have emerged, had he not been delivered by waking up? What inspires in Freud the fear of thinking? These questions will direct our analysis.

Many of Freud's dreams, as we have seen, deal unconsciously with the anguish born of Uncle Josef's crime. The dreams of the Uncle, Count Thun, *Non vixit,* Riding on a Horse, The Open-Air Closet, and the Botanical Monograph display the whole gamut of his unwitting nightly ruminations over Uncle Josef. The constant repetition of the same problem seems to indicate an unconscious effort at mastery, but one that ultimately fails. Freud remains chained to his uncle's dubious legacy, in part because he cannot admit to himself the silent pain and the profound upheaval it provoked.

This is why the attempt to dispose of his uncle's problem slides into subterfuge and wishful thinking in Freud's dreams. For example, the dream memorial to Josef bears the inscription *he did not live*. Freud also believes he is more fortunate than his friends because, after they die, he can have everything to himself alone. Moreover, should the dead dare to trouble him, just wait, he warns, he won't hesitate to blow them away with a piercing look. In any case, he has absolutely nothing to fear; his friends R. and N.—a simpleton and a criminal respectively, just like his uncle Josef—are the ones who need to beware; Sigmund Freud himself is beyond suspicion! Apart from the emotional denial, his endless ruminations about his uncle have yet another source. The Nightmare of Self-dissection will lead the way there, though without the dreamer's awareness. As a result, the nightmare shows us Freud's blocked self-analysis, giving a token of the obstructions he met on his way toward himself. The Nightmare of Self-dissection is a network of intertwined fragments Freud is utterly unable to disentangle. Yet they endure forever in his mind—like the living dead.

In most of Freud's dreams, Uncle Josef's presence is more or less directly identifiable. Not so in the Nightmare of Self-dissection. Is it because an essentially different problem is paramount? We do not think so. It is simply that another aspect of the events of 1865–1866 is being treated there, a more deeply hidden aspect because it is more dangerous. As a child, Freud must have been all too aware of his uncle's arrest and imprisonment, but there were other facets of the drama about which he did not have the faintest knowledge. The Austrian police minister's memorandum provides the decisive clue: "Two highly suspicious letters [were] sent from England by two sons . . . of a brother of Josef Freud's.

In one of these letters we are told that the brother's sons have as much money as there is sand by the sea . . . In another letter, they ask him . . . to find a bank for the merchandise where the turn-over would be larger, faster, and more profitable."

We assume that Freud had no conscious idea, as a child or at any time afterward, of the existence of these incriminating letters and of the suspicions they cast over his half-brothers. Did over-heard bits of conversation, haphazard looks, or gestures of an-guish in the family instill in Freud the fear of a greater danger than his uncle's conviction and imprisonment? The terrified tenor of his nightmare leads us to think so. The grown-ups' secret panic (perfectly comprehensible under the circumstances) over the compromising letters explains for us the difference between the Nightmare of Self-dissection and Freud's other dreams. If thus far we have been able to make progress with relative ease—in great measure using Freud's own interpretive techniques, such as dis-placements or condensations of meaning, homonyms and ho-mophony, ambiguity, and anagrams—the Nightmare of Self-dissection at first blush closes off all forms of access. Only after understanding the dream as an expression of Freud's very inability to dissect his mind like his pelvis will we be in a position to seize upon a handful of covert keys, scattered throughout the dream text and the accompanying associations. These keys will eventually open silence to speech.

On a first level of analysis, we perceive the indirect expression of Freud's unbridgeable difficulty in gaining insight into himself. This difficulty shows in the immediate consequences of his self-analytical operation and his thoughts relative to it. An initial impression of misleading freshness gives way to fatigue; the dreamer is quite unable to walk after the surgery he performs on his own body. First he hires a cab, then he has himself carried by a guide as they move over boggy terrain. Freud wonders in his associations "how much longer will my legs carry me?" He speaks of becoming "really frightened about my legs," a fear related to "perilous journeys" and to "an adventurous road that had scarcely ever been trodden before, leading into an undiscovered region."

The undiscovered region is of course none other than Freud himself; every commentator has agreed on this point. However, we are adding something new. Freud is a region where Freud himself cannot make headway. It is for this reason that his self-dissection throws him into both bodily and mental disarray. At first merely troubled, because deprived of his legs to embark on his self-exploration, Freud will end up being torn from his dream with a horror of thinking *(Gedankenschreck)*. In a final test, the dreamer finds himself before a chasm, but it proves to be impassable for lack of a practicable crossing. Unable to step into his inner self, Freud wakes up frightened. Yes, indeed, he cannot throw a bridge across the gulf, he cannot gain insight into the nightmarish abyss of his own family's life. What is the abyss? And if Freud cannot go there alone, who can serve as his guide?

In the preface to the second edition (1908) of *The Interpretation of Dreams,* Freud speaks of his book and self-analysis as having been undertaken in reaction to his father's death in 1896. In his final association to the Nightmare of Self-dissection, Freud also mentions a father's legacy before dying. Along with the documents about Uncle Josef's counterfeiting affair, we intend to use these pieces of information as interpretive clues. To analyze himself more fully, should Freud scrutinize his father's legacy? In the context of the nightmare, this would imply that Freud needs his father's help to cross the abyss yawning before him. "There the guide . . . laid two wooden boards . . . so as to bridge the chasm that had to be crossed . . . At that point I really became frightened about my legs." In the end Freud will stay at the edge of the precipice: to cross it, he would have to pass over "not the boards but children." At this idea he starts with horror. Who is the guide that proposes such an unsuitable crossing? Goethe's poetic lines, quoted in the associations—"The best of what you know, you cannot tell the boys"—suggest Freud's father. Did Jakob Freud take a silence to the grave? (Freud quotes these same lines by Goethe in the explanation to his Dream of the Uncle; I, 142).

Let us review the dream's central image of Freud's self-dissection. The *"task . . . related to a dissection of the lower part of my own body, my pelvis and legs . . . The pelvis had been eviscerated, and it was visible now in its superior, now in its inferior aspect, the two being mixed together. Thick flesh-coloured protuberances (which, in the dream itself, made me think of haemorrhoids) could be seen. Something which lay over it and was like crumpled silver-paper had also to be carefully fished out."* Aided by Freud's associations—"Louise N., the lady who was assisting me in my job in the dream, had been calling on me. 'Lend me something to read,' she had said . . . 'Have you nothing of your own?'"—we suspect that what needs to be dissected or read here, in this self-analytical operation, is Freud's own text, that is, the verbal body of his dream.

In point of fact, the crumpled *silver-paper*—to be "fished out," in the original German, to be carefully pieced together one by one (= *ausklauben*)—leads us to the like-sounding *syllable* (in German, silver = *Silber: Silbe* = syllable). Did the dream's syllables get crumpled or mixed up? Did the words describing Freud's self-dissection condense other words concerning his family's counterfeiting affair? The German names of the two bones that make up the pelvis, on which Freud chose to operate, are no doubt telling about Uncle Josef's impact on the family: a *cross* and a *shame* (sacrum = *Kreuz*bein: cross bone; innominate bone = *Scham*bein: shame bone). Freud's self-analytical operation seems to hover around these hidden thoughts. If, in this immediate context, we piece together the syllables describing Freud's self-dissection, they very closely approximate the words *false* or counterfeit *banknotes*. We interpret the German original as follows:

Freud operates on his legs = *Beine,* his pelvic *bone* = *Bein,* and *flesh*-colored = *fleisch*-rote = flesh red protuberances = *Kno*llen. These syllables yield bein-fleisch-kn-ote-n; unscrambled, they are nearly identical in pronunciation, through *fleisch: falsch* = false and *Bein: Ban,* to *f*a*lsche Ban-kn-ote-n* = *false* or *counterfeit bank notes.* These anagrammatic fragments are reinforced by association in the dream: (1) through the hemorrhoids because this image calls up piles or, in German, *knots: Hemorrhoidalknoten;* (2) through Freud's constant insistence on his problematic *legs* = *Beine* (Ban).

Forged notes, the *shame* and the *cross,* are the secret keys to Freud's self-dissection. They encourage us to interpret the next stage, "the road leading into an undiscovered region." Freud's uneasy progress on foot, his fatigue, his recurrent fear for his legs correspond to an attempted *forward movement of thought* that is yet tortured to the point of making him stop in horror. Freud's analysis of his inmost self, the adventurous journey leading to the undiscovered region, is an attempt to think about the "forged notes" and the "shame." We see the rest of the dream unfolding as follows: *Progressing in myself when it comes to my ancestors is far from easy. Nevertheless, I could make my self-analysis move forward, if only I dared. So, I took a cab, that is I dreamed the word* Waagen = *cab:* wagen = *to dare in order to pull myself along. It is immediately better this way. Still, there are spots where, the ground being slippery and boggy, my legs—my thoughts—refuse to move forward. I need a guide. With his help, I once again hope to make some headway within myself. But the guide sets me down at the edge of a precipice and now I am suddenly quite powerless to think any further. In vain does he put down two boards, undoubtedly to help me with some difficulty, to get me over to the next thought. Horrible, horrible! I just saw that the wooden planks were really children. I cannot go on thinking such thoughts. I woke up distraught, with a dread of thinking.*

What thought is unbearable for Freud? What is the abyss of thought that his guide—his father?—forbids him to cross? Is it the idea that Sigmund Freud's half-brothers in England, that is, his father's *children* from a first marriage, may somehow be tied to the shame of forged notes? The words that so startle Freud, *two boards* and *children,* suggest as much. If we turn to English— a language indicated by Rider Haggard's novel *She,* the book from which Freud says he borrowed the boards—the German original for *boards* = *Bretter* leads to the nearly homophonous English word *brethren.* (Note also that, in the police documents, Sigmund Freud's half-brothers in England are referred to as the "brother-sons" [*Brüdersöhne*] or the children of a brother [of Jakob Freud].)

Is it Freud's brothers' undiscovered history in England that Freud's father took to the grave? Is it his brothers' drama that Freud should absolutely never be allowed to see? Is this why he imagines himself buried (prior to thinking of the task he leaves to his own children) in an *Etruscan* tomb, a language that has remained undeciphered to this day? It would be useless to seek any direct answers. However, we do possess the indirect witness of Freud's dream.

In the associations to his Nightmare of Self-dissection, Freud refers to Rider Haggard's *She.* This novel, by an English author born in May 1856 like the dreamer, seems useful for describing Freud's psychological state, even though the summary he gives of it does not immediately suggest this kind of significance. Published in 1887, *She* tells of Leo Vincey's quest for a woman, who two thousand years earlier had slain her lover Kallikrates, Vincey's forebear, out of jealous spite. Vincey manages to find Ayesha, the murderer, but is unable to kill her, as his family legacy would demand, because, dazzled, he falls in love with her.

Ayesha is at present queen of the Tombs of Kor, a country whose inhabitants live in vast underground galleries, built once upon a time by an extinct people whose technique of embalming was far superior to that of the ancient Egyptians. The queen of Kor, attired like a mummy, lives as if buried alive at the heart of a volcano, in ceaseless vigil over the corpse of Kallikrates, her lover, dead for these two thousand years. Possessed of supernatural powers, she can make his body move but is unable to revive his soul. She keeps the corpse from disintegrating while she awaits the hour of her slain lover's resurrection. Taken aback by the facial resemblance between Vincey and Kallikrates, Ayesha believes she has been rewarded for her two thousand years of waiting. She takes Vincey to the flame of eternal life. As he hesitates, Ayesha enters the flame, and, under Vincey's terror-struck eyes, she dies, on her face the stamp of unutterable age. Vincey retraces his steps, over marshes and bottomless gulfs, bewildered, a victim of Ayesha's defunct beauty and bereft of all hope of ever fathoming her secret.

We believe that *She* has an important place in Freud's self-analytical dream because this novel tells of family situations that have remained long unsettled, as though buried alive. Most likely it is not so much the plot or the stories of adventure that have touched Freud. He must have been moved rather more by the description of a static world, in which age-old dramas forever hang in suspense, vainly awaiting a satisfactory resolution. In such a world, wholly given over to past calamities and oblivious to the present, nothing either truly lives or dies. This is why we see in *She*'s images of incompleteness and preservation, of entombment and embalming, the reflection of a permanently unresolved drama, the mark of an "encrypted" family trauma in Freud.

The Secret of Psychoanalysis

Like a dormant volcano, an old catastrophe smolders in Freud. A devastating eruption upset his childhood in 1865. Sowing despair, it interrupted life. The humiliation of an arrest, the fear of the consequences, the pall of suspicion cast over the entire family, all this abruptly altered the adults' behavior. Death in their sinking hearts, faces blank with despondency, the parents withdrew into a cocoon of silence. Nameless anguish blighted the whole family. Yesterday all was well, but fitful destiny turned it overnight. In the oppressive atmosphere of indefinable bewilderment, the child's questions quickly dried up. He found solace in his dreams. Thus the young Freud replaced his fallen, imprisoned uncle Josef with another Joseph from the Bible. That Joseph too went to prison, but through no fault of his own, and was later gloriously freed by the all-powerful Pharaoh himself, to become Pharaoh's indispensable right hand. This idealized image of a triumphant Joseph continued to guide the child even in his adult research, inspiring the forty-year-old author of *The Interpretation of Dreams.* In reality, however, the crushing weight of the calamity and the adults' secretiveness all but benumbed the young Freud: the true intensity of his family trauma never dawned on him.

Notwithstanding this personal background, or perhaps because of it, Freud advocated early on the necessity of knowing himself as a prerequisite for understanding others. Thus he undertook his self-analysis in the mid-1890s, trying to learn about his own unconscious, analyzing his dreams, slips of the tongue, recollections, and associations. At first systematically, later rather more episodically, he pursued his much admired self-exploration to the end of his life. Yet, no matter how thorough, Freud's self-analysis had to remain incomplete. The adults' shame quashed the family drama. Like the young Freud, the adult could never penetrate the wall of silence his family had erected around a catastrophe they considered unspeakable.

Freud undoubtedly knew at the time (1865–1866) about the mere fact of his uncle's arrest and conviction. He says as much in his autobiographical Dream of the Uncle with the Yellow Beard. However, he saw nothing of the havoc the calamity had worked upon him in the midst of his ravaged family. The extent of his trauma escaped Freud because he had no one to turn to. Amid the general affliction, who thinks of reassuring the children? On the contrary, the Freud family had to keep its troubles and anxieties from the children. It would have been dangerous for the whole family if any of the children had learned about the Austrian authorities' grave suspicions of Sigmund's half-brothers, Philip and Emmanuel. The grown-ups must have thought it necessary to shield the children from the fear that, following Josef's indictment for passing counterfeit rubles, the whole Freud family might be ruined. In this kind of anxiety-stricken and necessarily deceitful atmosphere, the child is left with little more than confusion, perhaps a vaguely felt though entirely mute question: What will become of me and of my desperate family?

The adults' obstinate silence aggravates the family catastrophe for children. A creeping form of bewilderment overcomes them, leading to a paradoxical and exceptionally painful emotional situation. Notwithstanding the disaster's diffuse and constantly oppressive presence, its essential details dwindle before the children's inquiring eyes. When the adults compound a family trauma with silence, children are forever denied insight, even after they have grown up. In such a constellation, children have only one choice, to keep their anguish and gnawing suspicions to themselves, carefully shutting them up in an inner safe or psychic tomb. This is why Freud's self-analysis had to remain by definition incomplete. His sincerest desire to know himself met with the fear of seeing himself bend under the yoke of a suppressed family trauma. His genuine desire to understand himself faded in the face of his own unsettling and unformulated questions. For Freud the outcome proved to be a trap: he carried out his self-analysis with the secret promise that he would ask no questions about his family's murky past.

This is the heartbeat of our hypothesis. Freud's darkness about himself put him at odds with his research. Unable to know himself and his family because of a secret family disaster, he placed obstacles in the way of knowing others. Freud, the inventor of psychoanalysis, is the architect of a paradox: he is perfectly willing to look for the causes of mental suffering so long as what he finds will obey his control. Freud's flawed methods of investigation derive from his need to foresee his results. Willy-nilly, his radical psychoanalytic discoveries (about the unconscious, dreams, psychosexuality, and the mechanisms of symptom formation) led to a predictable system of identifying universal sources of psychic turmoil. Because of a foggy family disaster, partially explained and partially concealed, Freud vacillated. He would perhaps have liked nothing more than to clear up his family's drama, but, at the same time, butting against immovable obstacles, he thwarted his own inquiry. Thus, while Freud invented entirely original and highly flexible procedures of discovery, he also locked them into a framework that shackled them, defeating his ideal of unbiased research.

Despite Freud's extraordinary advances in the field of human psychology, his family's drama forever remained out of reach. For this reason, both Freudian psychoanalysis and Sigmund Freud became self-contradictory. Of course, the idea of psychoanalysis ultimately implied the possibility of understanding his own and his loved ones' pain. Yet Freud's enterprise could not help falling into the trap of his family's concealments. As a result, Freud worked tirelessly against his inmost ambition, the freedom to investigate the mind. Freudian theory keeps generating internal oppositions, forcing its most original procedures of discovery into predetermined directions, because Freud conducted his psychological research against the backdrop of a permanent and compulsory blindness about his own family's life.

The young Freud's silent pain and the contradictions of Freudian psychoanalysis have the same root, *a trauma of inaccessibility,* stemming from the prohibition against asking questions, from the impossibility of knowing. Freud preserved, in himself and at the core of his theory, a basic upheaval because he could never speak freely with anyone about his family catastrophe; thus he could never overcome it, be consoled, or be truly purged of it.

Conclusion

We have questioned Freud because we have discovered that, from the beginning, he thwarted the progress of psychoanalysis by adopting contradictory and self-defeating methodologies. We have wanted an answer to the question: Why is it that in Freudian ideas and practices extraordinary openness is so often overpowered by deaf-minded unreceptiveness? The hope of reaching into the furthest recesses of the psyche did guide Freud's efforts throughout his career. So we acclaim him whenever he urges and accomplishes the removal of repressive censorship, when he tears down our emotional, intellectual, or sexual prisons. But should we follow him when he shuts the very doors that, in the face of much resistance and hostility, he has single-handedly pried open?

Our ultimate goal is to safeguard only those aspects of Freud's work which truly allowed him to see the mind and resolve emotional turmoil. That is why we began by isolating the source of a hitherto unnoticed yet fundamental confusion in psychoanalysis:

its founder, Sigmund Freud, simultaneously fostered and frustrated unprejudiced psychological inquiry. Still, the attacks upon psychoanalysis that would brand it a quasi-religion, deceptively dressed in pseudo-scientific garb, seem to us futile, because the Freud bashers of today and yesterday categorically refuse to consider the genuine achievement of his research into the workings of the human mind.

We are, of course, just as distrustful of those who would see in psychoanalysis a set of ready-made keys. These people are fatally blind to the theoretical, clinical, and institutional contradictions that have torn psychoanalysis asunder. We have chosen "the golden middle"—relentless criticism combined with certainty about the *inherent potential* of psychoanalysis. It is our duty henceforth to avoid perpetuating the traps of Freudianism and to nurture, with the fiercest of scrutinies, the true genius of Freud's authentic discoveries. At present this implies a complete transformation of the field of psychoanalysis.

Notes

Index

Notes

Introduction

1. This book stems from research begun in 1977, and is based in part on Maria Torok's more than three decades of psychoanalytic practice and theoretical work. See Nicolas Abraham and Maria Torok, *The Wolf Man's Magic Word*, ed. and trans. Nicholas Rand (Minneapolis: University of Minnesota Press, 1986); idem, *The Shell and the Kernel: Renewals of Psychoanalysis*, vol. 1, ed. and trans. Nicholas Rand (Chicago: University of Chicago Press, 1994); Nicolas Abraham, *Jonas* (Paris: Flammarion, 1981); *Rhythms: On the Work, Translation, and Psychoanalysis*, collected and presented by Nicholas Rand and Maria Torok, trans. Benjamin Thigpen and Nicholas Rand (Palo Alto: Stanford University Press, 1995). These works, written and originally published between 1959 and 1975, have renewed both the theory and the practice of psychoanalysis in France. For background information see N. Rand, "Introduction: Renewals of Psychoanalysis," in Abraham and Torok, *The Shell and the Kernel*, pp. 1–22.

I. Fundamental Contradictions of Freudian Thought

1. Nicolas Abraham seems to us to have solved this problem implicitly by granting legitimacy to nothing but the psychoanalysis of unique specificities, both on the level of the individual and the level of collective or historical situations. He characterized universal forms

of psychoanalytic interpretation with fixed codes as mere pseudo-analytic misapprehension. See Abraham and Torok, *The Shell and the Kernel,* vol. 1, and "Le symbole ou l'au-delà du phénomène" (1961), forthcoming in English translation in *The Shell,* vol. 2.

2. We consider neither Freud's announcement of his rejection of the seduction theory nor his gradual adoption of the Oedipus complex as a definitive resolution of this question; see below.

3. In *The Assault on Truth: Freud's Suppression of the Seduction Theory* (New York: Farrar, Straus, and Giroux, 1984), J. M. Masson argues that after September 1897 Freud hesitated briefly over his disavowal of the seduction theory but that—despite his better judgment—he abandoned it because he feared the theory might impede his professional success. We cannot corroborate this thesis, especially since Masson's own annotated edition of *The Complete Letters of Sigmund Freud to Wilhelm Fliess* points in a completely different direction. The letters show clearly that even in 1900 Freud was far from repudiating his earlier theory. The notes in the earlier, expurgated edition of this correspondence, *The Origins of Psychoanalysis: Letters to Wilhelm Fliess* (1954), and Ernst Kris's introduction sought to validate Freud's claim that he had swiftly repudiated the seduction theory; this validation led to the censorship of letters and passages indicating the opposite.

II. Psychoanalysis in the Eye of Literature

1. Jensen's *Gradiva* (1903) has long been out of print in English and is not included in the *Standard Edition.* Only Philip Rieff's edition of *Delusion and Dream and Other Essays* (also out of print) carries both Jensen's text and Freud's commentary. German and French speakers have easier access in currently available paperback editions.

2. See also Freud's influential essays of literary and aesthetic criticism: *The Theme of the Three Caskets* (1913), *The Uncanny* (1919), and *Dostoevsky and Patricide* (1928).

3. Similarly Freud used E. T. A. Hoffmann's *The Sandman* as a literary case study to illustrate the psychoanalytic concept of the castration complex. See our essay "'The Sandman' Looks at 'The Uncanny,'" in *Speculations after Freud: Psychoanalysis, Philosophy and Culture,*

ed. Sonu Shamdasani and Michael Münchow (London: Routledge, 1994), pp. 185–204.

4. Philip Rieff aptly remarks in his introduction to Freud's essay on *Gradiva:* "Freud found the world of the literary imagination entirely submissive. Jensen might resist. But like a hat or any other prop on the stage of universal meanings, Jensen's leading character allows his unconscious to be undressed with the greatest of ease . . . The fictional character becomes the ideally docile patient of psychoanalysis." He later adds: "Freud systematically treated an entire piece of fiction, transforming *Gradiva,* by means of his voracious interpretive method, from an anticipation of psychoanalytic truth into an illustration of it." Sigmund Freud, *Delusion and Dream and Other Essays,* ed. Philip Rieff (Boston: Beacon Press, 1956), pp. 3, 7.

5. The literature on *Gradiva* is sparse. Scholars have sought to expand the scope of the Freudian interpretation by bringing to bear on it ideas Freud was to develop subsequently (see Bellemin-Noël, Kofman, Roger) or by isolating elements in the story that might lend themselves to Lacanian rather than Freudian concepts (see Ackerman). Others have examined the German literary and philosophical traditions that inform the works of both Jensen and Freud (see Favier, Haag, Henninger). Jan Ackerman, *"Delusions and Dreams:* Freud's Pompeian Love Letter," in Vera J. Camden, ed., *Compromise Formations: Current Directions in Psychoanalytic Criticism* (Kent, Ohio: Kent State University Press, 1989), pp. 45–59; Jean Bellemin-Noël, *Gradiva au pied de la lettre* (Paris: PUF, 1983); Georges Favier, "Freud lecteur de Jensen," *Cahiers d'Etudes Germaniques,* 10 (1986), pp. 55–107; Ingrid Haag, "La *Gradiva* de Jensen" ibid., pp. 109–121; Peter Henninger, "Autour de la *Gradiva,*" ibid., pp. 123–149; Sarah Kofman, *Quatre romans analytiques* (Paris: Galilée, 1973); Max Milner, *Freud et l'interprétation de la littérature* (Paris: SEDES, 1980); Alain Roger, *Hérésies du désir* (Seyssel: Champ Vallon, 1985).

6. Norbert indicates his transitional state at one point by calling the young woman Zoe-Gradiva. At the close of his emotional maturation, that is, by the end of the tale, he gives up the temporary name Gradiva altogether.

7. The idea of the illness of mourning was first introduced by Maria Torok in 1968. See "The Illness of Mourning and the Fantasy of

the Exquisite Corpse," in Abraham and Torok, *The Shell and the Kernel*, vol. 1, pp. 107–124.

8. In this respect Freud follows Jensen's text. "Fräulein Zoe, the embodiment of cleverness and clarity, makes her own mind quite transparent to us" (DDJ, 33). However, Freud's idea of Zoe as a psychoanalyst is totally alien to the story.

9. In Norbert Hanold's case it is not appropriate to speak of a psychoanalytic cure but rather of a spontaneous and personal triumph over his illness of mourning. His emotional recovery combines renewed interest in life with a gradual awakening to sexuality. His unexpected encounter with Zoe focuses his long-budding sexual desires. Indeed, his emotional readiness to love a woman is the prerequisite for the spectacular change that comes over Norbert in just a few days; he quickly relinquishes the idea of the dead rising from the grave and proposes to wed the truly vivacious Zoe.

10. It is not at all uncommon for Freud to alter his earlier interpretations in the light of subsequent theories. A clear case in point is his reevaluation, in terms of the death drive, of Emmy von N.'s case from the *Studies in Hysteria* (1895) in a footnote he added in 1924. Freud's new theory on mourning did not produce a similar return to Jensen's *Gradiva*. Actually, Freud chose to restate his analogy between repression and the fate of Pompeii as late as 1937 in his essay *Constructions in Analysis*. Had he wished to do so, he certainly could have modified the analogy in terms of mourning after 1915.

11. See Norbert's interest in the ancient relief of a woman (Gradiva) whose life, catastrophic death, and burial he situates in Pompeii; his trip to Pompeii to discover a trace of her; Gradiva's "ghostly" visitation in Pompeii and her meetings with the young man who is now convinced of Pompeii's spontaneous revival; his discovery of love with Zoe in Pompeii; his wish to take his wedding trip to Pompeii.

12. "Our views on repression, on the genesis of delusions and allied disorders, on the formation and solution of dreams, on the part played by erotic life, and on the methods by which such disorders are cured, are far from being the common property of science, let alone the assured possession of educated people" (DDJ, 90–91). "When, from the year 1893 onwards, I plunged into investigations such as these of the origin of mental disorders, it would certainly never have occurred to me to look for confirmation of my findings

in imaginative writings. I was thus more than a little surprised to find that the author of *Gradiva*, which was published in 1903, had taken as the basis of its creation the very thing that I believed myself to have freshly discovered" (DDJ, 54). Freud points to one of two explanations for the allegedly exceptional convergence between his own views and Jensen's *Gradiva*. Either Jensen knew Freud's theories without quoting them, or they both recognized the same universal laws of mental functioning.

III. Transmissions of Psychoanalysis

1. For a more complete discussion of the case study of Emmy von N. see Maria Torok, "A Remembrance of Things Deleted: Between Sigmund Freud and Emmy von N.," in Abraham and Torok, *The Shell and the Kernel*, pp. 234–248.
2. Here is another excerpt, from a letter by Freud to Jones (quoted from AT, 181) dated 29 May 1933: "[Mrs. Severn] seems to have produced in him a *pseudologica phantastica*, since he believed her accounts of the most strange childhood traumas, which he then defended against us."
3. Although Freud certainly deserves criticism for his attitude after Ferenczi's death, it is important to know that, in their correspondence during the period 1929–1932, Freud did his best to save their personal if not their theoretical friendship. In short, Freud never rejected Ferenczi as a person; he swore off the thinker who came to disagree with him.
4. On the concepts of preservative repression, intrapsychic crypts, and family secrets that are unwittingly handed down to descendants, see the writings of Nicolas Abraham and Maria Torok between 1968 and 1975 as collected in *The Wolf Man's Magic Word* and *The Shell and the Kernel*, vol. 1.

IV. Gaining Insight into Freud

1. Accompanied by Barbro Sylwan, Maria Torok consulted the original documents in 1977 in the National Police Archives in Vienna. For additional details, the reader can consult a number of related documents, transcribed and commented on (often with a gratuitously accusatory twist) by the historian Renée Gicklhorn in *Sigmund*

Freud und der Onkeltraum [Sigmund Freud and the Uncle Dream] (Vienna: Eigenverlag, 1976); Alain de Mijolla, "Mein Onkel Josef à la une!" *Etudes Freudiennes* 15–16 (1979): 183–192; Marianne Krüll, *Freud and His Father;* a detailed summary of some documents is also available in Alexander Grinstein, *Freud at the Crossroads* (Madison, Conn.: International Universities Press, 1990), pp. 67–72.

2. Didier Anzieu, *L'Auto-analyse de Freud et la découverte de la psychanalyse* (Paris: PUF, 1959, 1975); Edith Buxbaum, "Freud's Dream Interpretation in Light of His Letters to Fliess," *Bulletin of the Menninger Clinic* 15 (1951): 197–212; Ernst Kris, "Introduction to the Letters to Wilhelm Fliess," in Freud, *The Origins of Psycho-Analysis: Letters to Wilhelm Fliess, Drafts and Notes, 1887–1902,* ed. Marie Bonaparte, Anna Freud, and Ernst Kris (London: Hogarth Press, 1954), pp. 3–47. See also Heinz Schott, *Zauberspiegel der Seele: Freud und die Geschichte der Selbstanalyse* [The Soul and Its Magical Mirror: Freud and the History of Self-Analysis] (Vandenhoek Ruprecht, 1985); this work contains a substantial bibliography of European and American scholarship on the subject; in the United States the standard work is the collection edited by Mark Kanzer and Jules Glenn, *Freud and His Self-Analysis* (New York: Norton, 1979).

3. Wladimir Granoff, *Filiations* (Paris: Minuit, 1975); Alexander Grinstein, *On Sigmund Freud's Dreams* (Detroit: Wayne State University Press, 1968); Conrad Stein, "Rome imaginaire: Fragment d'un commentaire de *L'Interprétation des rêves,* de Sigmund Freud," *L'Inconscient* 1 (1967): 1–30; idem, "L'identification à Freud dans l'auto-analyse," *L'Inconscient* 7 (1968): 99–114; see scattered remarks in Octave Mannoni, *Freud* (Paris: Seuil, 1968), and the collection of German essays edited by Jürgen von Scheidt, *Der Unbekannte Freud* (Frankfurt: Fischer, 1987).

4. In R. D. Loewenstein, ed., *Psychoanalysis: A General Psychology* (New York: International Universities Press, 1966), pp. 45–85.

5. Abraham and Torok reinterpreted the Wolf Man's case with the hypothesis that his family forced him to conceal a sexual secret; see *The Wolf Man's Magic Word.* Abraham and Torok also described their discoveries on family secrets in parts 3 and 4 of *The Shell and the Kernel.*

6. Representative work by Maria Torok includes "L'Os de la fin: quelques jalons pour l'étude du *verbarium* freudien," *Cahiers Confrontation* 1 (1979): 163–186; "What Is Occult in Occultism: Between Sigmund Freud and Sergei Pankeiev, Wolf Man," in Abraham and Torok, *The Wolf Man's Magic Word*, pp. 84–106; "La correspondance Ferenczi-Freud," *Cahiers Confrontations* 12 (1984): 79–99; "Unpublished by Freud to Fliess: Restoring an Oscillation," *Critical Inquiry* 12 (Winter 1986): 391–398; "A Remembrance of Things Deleted," in Abraham and Torok, *The Shell and the Kernel*, pp. 234–248; with Rand, "The Secret of Psychoanalysis: History Reads Theory," in *The Trial(s) of Psychoanalysis*, ed. Françoise Meltzer (Chicago: University of Chicago Press), pp. 65–73; "La psychanalyse devant son secret," in Nicholas Rand, *Le Cryptage et la vie des oeuvres: Etude du secret dans les textes* (Paris: Aubier, 1989), pp. 147–162; "'The Sandman' Looks at 'The Uncanny': Hoffmann's Question to Freud," in *Speculations after Freud*, ed. Shamdasani and Münchow, pp. 185–204. See also Barbro Sylwan, "Le ferd-ikt: lettre ouverte au professeur Freud, dédiée à l'oeuvre de Nicolas Abraham," *Etudes Freudiennes* 13–14 (1978): 127–174; and idem, "Freud and Co., marchands de Manchester: A propos de la mort de Philipp Freud et ses effets," *Cahiers Confrontation* 18 (1987): 145–158.

7. Several scholars, among them Alexander Grinstein in *On Sigmund Freud's Dreams* and Didier Dumas in *L'Ange et le fantôme* (Paris: Minuit, 1985), isolate the death of Julius, a baby brother of Freud's, as the principal trauma of his life.

8. As regards the dream's date and its possible relationship to Josef Freud's death, Grinstein puts forward the same hypothesis in *Freud at the Crossroads*, p. 65.

9. Freud himself calls attention, albeit indirectly, to the uncle-nephew relationship as involving either Josef and himself or himself and John. "In the dream of my uncle which I have just mentioned, the antithetical, affectionate affect probably arose from an infantile source . . . , for the uncle-nephew relationship, owing to . . . earliest experiences of my childhood . . . had become the source of all my friendships and all my hatreds" (I, 472).

10. We agree with Didier Anzieu's suspicion that these two dreams are contemporaneous.

Index

Index

Index

Narcissism, 36
National Police Archives (Vienna), 231n1
Neuroses, 12, 25, 27, 29–30, 33, 35, 38, 40–42, 118, 143–144, 158
Non Vixit, Dream of, 172, 183–193
"Norbert Hanold," 55–57, 59–75, 77, 81–93

Objective reality, 25, 28, 38–44
Obsessions, 12
Oedipus complex, 4, 35, 52, 117, 134, 158, 162
Open-Air Closet, Dream of the, 172, 197–201, 206
Ovid: *Metamorphoses,* 58

Paneth, Josef, 191–192
Parental intercourse, observation of, 25, 41
Patricide, 44
Penis envy, 4
Phobias, 12
Pompeii, 55–74, 78–93
Prehistoric reality, 41
Primal scenes, 41, 158
Proper names, forgetting of, 158
Psychical reality, 5, 24–44
Psychoanalysis: paradoxes/contradictions in, ix-x, 1–6, 48, 76–77, 80–81, 97, 107–108, 134–135, 141–143, 145, 164, 221–224; changing attitudes toward, ix-x, 6; internal destructive power of, x; indefensible aspects of, x-xi; future of, xi; methodological flaws in, 3, 5–6, 76, 139–144; significance of Freudian thought, 4, 47; of literature, 5, 48–94; renewal of, 5–6, 224; dream interpretation, 9–23, 90–93; psychical reality, 24–44; truth versus falsehood, 25–29, 35–43; applied, 50, 52–53, 93–94, 144; distortions caused by, 54, 76–94; historical topography of, 97–107; transmission of, 97–99, 105;

and catharsis, 108–114; and constructive criticism, 115–135; genesis of, 139–140, 142; secret of, 219–222
Psychosexual development, 4, 36
Pygmalion myth, 58

Rabelais, François, 199
Rank, Otto, 106
Reality, 5, 24–44, 105, 117–118, 121–122, 132, 143
Repression, 5, 14, 49, 51–52, 54–57, 66–67, 77–88, 93, 134, 144
Riding on a Horse, Dream of, 172, 193–197
Rieff, Philip, 229n4
Rousseau, Jean-Jacques: *Confessions,* 159

Sachs, Hans, 106
Schliemann, Heinrich, 32
Schur, Max: *Freud: Living and Dying,* 160–161, 163–164
Screen memories, 34–35, 202
Secrets, 160–162, 164–165, 168–171, 218, 220–222, 232n5
Seduction theory, 5, 25–37, 42, 48, 102–104, 122, 132–133, 161–162
Self-Dissection, Dream of, 172, 208–218
Sexual desire. *See* Desire
Sexual fantasies, 25–37
Sexuality, 4, 35, 51–52, 158, 162
Sexual material in dreams, 10, 12–13, 17–18
Sexual repression, 5, 49, 51–52, 54–57, 66–67, 77, 82–83, 87–88, 93, 144
Sexual traumas, 25–37, 42, 102–104, 123–132
Stein, Conrad, 159
Stekel, Wilhelm, 13
Strachey, James, 174
Superego, 36, 117, 134